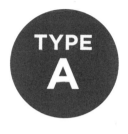

TYPE
A

Eat Right 4 Your Type

PERSONALIZED COOKBOOK

TYPE
A

Eat Right 4
Your Type

PERSONALIZED COOKBOOK

**150+ Healthy Recipes
for Your Blood Type Diet®**

Dr. Peter J. D'Adamo
with Kristin O'Connor

Photographs by Kristin O'Connor

Previously published as *Personalized Living
Using the Blood Type Diet® (Type A)*

B

BERKLEY BOOKS, NEW YORK

THE BERKLEY PUBLISHING GROUP
Published by the Penguin Group
Penguin Group (USA) LLC
375 Hudson Street, New York, New York 10014, USA

USA | Canada | UK | Ireland | Australia | New Zealand | India | South Africa | China

Penguin Books Ltd., Registered Offices: 80 Strand, London WC2R 0RL, England
For more information about the Penguin Group, visit penguin.com.

PUBLISHING HISTORY
Previously published in eBook format as *Personalized Living Using the Blood Type Diet®* *(Type A)* by Drum Hill Publishing, LLC in 2012
Berkley trade paperback edition: October 2013

Library of Congress Cataloging-in-Publication Data

D'Adamo, Peter J.
Eat right 4 your type personalized cookbook type A : 150+ healthy recipes for your blood type diet / Dr. Peter J. D'Adamo with Kristin O'Connor ; photographs by Kristin O'Connor.
    p. cm.
ISBN 978-0-425-26945-9 (pbk.)
 1. Diet therapy. 2. Nutrition. 3. Blood groups. 4. Naturopathy. I. O'Connor, Kristin.
II. Title. III. Title: Eat right for your type personalized cookbook type A.
  RM219.D288 2013
  641.5'631—dc23
                          2013021050

PRINTED IN THE UNITED STATES OF AMERICA

10   9   8   7   6   5

Cover design by Jason Gill
Cover photo by Christopher Bierlein
Book design by Pauline Neuwirth

Contents

Type A v

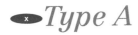 *Type A*

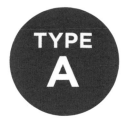

TYPE
A

Eat Right 4
Your Type

PERSONALIZED COOKBOOK

Introduction

Let food be thy medicine,

and medicine be thy food.

—HIPPOCRATES

FOOD HAS THE potential to heal and strengthen our physical bodies, support our recovery from injury and illness, and potentially change our genetic destinies.

Not only does food provide sustenance and nourishment, it provides an opportunity for creative expression and community, whether it is in developing new recipes or ways to prepare a certain food or in sharing a meal with others. When I wrote *Eat Right 4 Your Type* in 1996, I explored the connections between blood type and diet, and outlined specific nutritional programs for each blood type. Since it was published fifteen years ago, I have continued to research and write about the role that foods play in our lives, and I have tried to create support materials and guidance for people who follow the Blood Type Diet.

In 1998, I wrote *Cook Right 4 Your Type*, which acted as a handbook for my readers, providing recipes, cooking tips, and planning guidelines to help navigate the process of food planning and preparation. I always wanted to take this further as I felt there was an aesthetic quality about food and food preparation that should be reflected in a book, not just with great recipes but also with beautiful, four-color photography that celebrates food. About three years ago, I met Kristin O'Connor. Although she came to see me as a patient, our conversation turned to following the Blood Type Diet, cooking, food preparation, and the work she was doing as a personal chef, food stylist, and food blogger.

I was impressed by her dedication to nutrition and healthy eating and by her ability to simplify the food preparation process, which for some people can be quite daunting. Over the ensuing months as we worked together as doctor and patient, our conversations returned again and again to food. I felt that I had found in Kristin the perfect person to collaborate on a book project that would blend the scientific concepts of the Blood Type Diet with the artistry of cooking to create a visually stunning cookbook specifically designed for each blood type. Kristin has a passion for the Blood Type Diet that is unparalleled and an encyclopedic knowledge of the food lists for each of the blood types. She is creative and resourceful, and she appreciates and respects the need for food to both taste delicious and be nourishing.

For the past year, I have been enjoying the recipes included in the books, and I have to say that I've been knocked out by how delicious they are. They are also easy to prepare, as I know most of us have limited hours in the day for food planning and preparation. The recipes contained in these books are suitable for an individual and for families, as well as for special events and entertaining. Additionally, there are helpful food preparation tips, suggestions for how to organize your kitchen, food storage guidelines, and suggested resources that can make meal planning and preparation easier. My goal has always been to provide accessible information that is easy to incorporate into daily life, and I believe that Kristin has accomplished this.

These cookbooks represent new food and healthy lifestyle possibilities for my readers; they combine the science behind the Blood Type Diet with Kristin's expertise not only as a chef but as a believer and follower of these concepts, and packages them in a beautiful, four-color format. The recipes contained within are appropriate for your blood type and compliant with the food lists, and they are delicious and made with love—love of food, love of health, and love of sharing this with others on both Kristin's and my part.

I invite you to join us on the continued journey of personalized living. I am confident that you will find a trusted companion in these cookbooks, one who will make your life richer and healthier as you experiment with the recipes that were developed specifically to be right for your type.

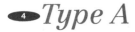

Type A at a Glance

PEACEFUL. IT IS the best adjective I can think of to describe the Type A diet and lifestyle, essentially maintaining balance in life through a mostly vegetarian diet; light, relaxing exercise; and eating frequent small meals. I'm sure 99 percent of you live a much different life; one in the real world with busy schedules and possibly little time for relaxation. Not to fear, eating and living as a Type A in our fast-paced world is certainly achievable with a little guidance. Let's start with what to eat.

Type As thrive on a diet full of soy protein, fresh vegetables, whole grains, and fruits. To enhance the effects of this primarily vegetarian diet, it is best to eat these foods in their most natural state: fresh and organic. This is not to say that you cannot eat any animal proteins, both chicken and turkey are *Neutrals*, which means that eating them once in a while will provide your body with added protein and not harm you, but they are not foods that promote health for Type A. Cod, salmon, whitefish, and trout are a few examples of seafood that are *Beneficial*, while there are several more that are *Neutral* to Type A, adding diversity to a typical vegetarian diet.

Eating for health and weight loss for Type A are truly intertwined. One of the health issues common for As is an overly sensitive immune system as well as a propensity for a greater reaction to stress. When our bodies feel stress in any form, whether it is through exercise, emotional highs and lows, or pressure at work, the physiological response is an increase in the stress hormone cortisol. When functioning properly, cortisol levels are the highest in the morning and decrease throughout the day. Type As, however, are prone to elevated levels of cortisol, which disrupts blood sugar and creates susceptibility toward diabetes (types I and II). In an effort to maintain blood sugar balance, it is essential for As to eat small meals more frequently during the day. Reducing cortisol levels will also result in weight loss. If you have ever seen advertisements that talk about weight-loss pills that reduce cortisol and thus reduce fat, especially around the belly, then this might be ringing a bell for you. Luckily, you do not

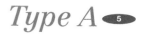

need to run out and buy pills because you now have the secret . . . the Blood Type Diet.

The Blood Type Diet has taken personalized nutrition to a higher level with the introduction of the influence Secretor Status has on our health. Approximately 80 percent of the population are Secretors, which means that the majority of us secrete our blood-type antigens in our bodily fluids such as saliva and mucus. As I explain in *Live Right 4 Your Type*:

> Subtyping your blood, especially your Secretor Status, provides an even greater specificity of identification. Your blood type doesn't just sit inert in your body. It is expressed in countless ways . . . A simple analogy would be a faucet. Depending on the water pressure, the faucet might pour or dribble . . . In the same way, your Secretor Status relates to how much and where your blood type antigen is expressed in your body.

Being a Secretor means that you can immediately attack viruses, bacteria, and other foreign bodies as they come in contact with your body, through secretions in your saliva. Non-Secretors do not have this first line of defense; however, their internal defenses are more powerful than Secretors. All of this means that there are some foods that are suitable for Secretors that may not be for Non-Secretors (NS) and vice versa. To address this, we have tagged all recipes in this book that are appropriate for Non-Secretors, and when possible, substitutions are provided to make the other recipes acceptable and healthful for Non-Secretors.

Reducing stress is obviously more than what you eat. Especially in a world with excessive stimulation, noise, crowds, and busy lives, it is important to make stress reduction a priority if not a daily habit. There are relaxation DVDs to listen to, yoga classes or tapes, meditation techniques readily available online, and new forms of calming exercise popping up all the time. The tools are out there; it's up to you to figure out what works for your lifestyle and interests.

In this book, you will find recipes, menus, and tools specifically designed for your Type A diet and Secretor Status. Please refer to your SWAMI© Personalized Nutrition Software Program guide if you have one (SWAMI is a proprietary software program designed to produce a unique, one-of-a-kind diet protocol based on your blood type, a series of biometric measurements, and your personal history. For more information, see page 234 in the Appendix). The goal is to make life easier for you once you begin your Blood Type Diet, so dive in and enjoy.

First Things First

Beneficial Foods

Here is a list of basics to keep in your kitchen with the thought that there will be times when meals have to be spontaneous. If you have essentials from your *Beneficial* and *Neutral* lists on hand, no matter what you make, it will be something good for you.

Let's Start with the Fridge

Salad Base

Pick your favorite greens or mix it up each time you go to the grocery store, keeping these salad base options in mind:

Chicory	Red leaf lettuce	Spinach
Escarole	Romaine	

This will give you a great start to a last-minute salad or an added crunch to a sandwich.

Roasted Vegetables

The best thing you can do for yourself is to keep hearty, fresh vegetables on hand to roast for dinner, make in bulk to add to your last-minute salad the next day, or add to a frittata for breakfast. Roasted vegetables are a terrific leftover to keep on hand. Most vegetables work well when tossed with olive oil and sea salt and roasted in a 375 degree oven for 12 to 20 minutes (depending on the size and density of the vegetables). Here are a few that are both *Beneficial* to Type A and take well to roasting:

 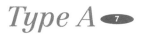

BENEFICIALS

Artichoke hearts	Kale
Broccoli	Onion
Broccolini	Parsnip
Carrots	Pumpkin
Fennel	

NEUTRALS

Asparagus	Celeriac
Beets	Rutabaga
Brussels sprouts	Squash
Cauliflower	Zucchini

Keeping a few of these vegetables in your fridge each week will come in handy and is a perfect way to add more *Beneficials* to your diet.

Fruit

Fruit is a perfect snack paired with nuts or nut butters, but you can also use fruit to make desserts or add dried fruit to cereal or salads. Some fruits even work well in savory dishes.

BENEFICIALS

Apricots	
Blackberries	Grapefruit
Blueberries	Lemons
Boysenberries	Limes
Cherries	Pineapple
Cranberries	Plums
Figs (Dried)	Prunes

Milk

Although Type As are not allowed cow milk, alternative milks are great to have on hand for smoothies, cereal, some soups, and baked goods. Acceptable milk options for you as Type A:

BENEFICIALS	NEUTRALS
Soy Milk	Rice Milk
	Almond Milk

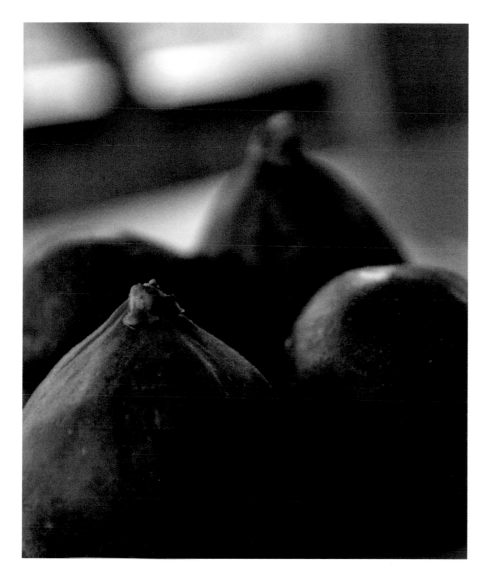

Extras

What about those things we all have hanging around in the door of our fridge like salad dressings, condiments, and relishes? Toss out those chemical-heavy bottles and jars and replace them with fresh and tasty homemade versions. Here are a few things that will save your taste buds from boredom:

Carrot-Ginger Dressing **NS** *
Citrus Dressing **NS** *
Fresh herbs: basil, oregano, parsley, thyme

Ghee
Ground flaxseeds
Herb Dressing NS *
Lemons
Olive Oil/Light Olive Oil

*Recipes provided in the book

Protein

The Type A diet is based on vegetable proteins, hearty grains, and fresh, pure fruits and vegetables. That said, maintaining a balance of protein, carbohydrates, and healthy fat in your diet is still essential. Understanding where to find vegetable proteins may be a new adventure for you, so below is a list to get you started. Try to diversify your sources of protein, just as you would if you remained a meat eater. Not many people eat beef every night for dinner, so try not to stick to one kind of protein here. You can add a few *Neutrals* to this list, but focus on the *Beneficials* as often as possible.

Please note that it is recommended that all poultry be organic and all beef be grass fed and organic.

BENEFICIALS
Soy (soy cheese, soy milk, tempeh, tofu)
Beans (adzuki, black, black-eyed peas, fava, lentils, soybeans, pinto)
Nuts (peanuts, walnuts)
Nut butters (peanut butter—*Beneficial* or almond butter—*Neutral*). Almond butter is inexpensive and easily found in supermarkets or natural food stores. If your SWAMI personalized nutrition plan indicates one type of nut that is *Beneficial* above the rest, use that one and make your own butter in the food processor.
Seafood (carp, cod, mackerel, monkfish, perch, pickerel, pollack, red snapper, salmon, sardine, snail, trout, whitefish, whiting)

NEUTRALS
Cheeses (mozzarella, feta, goat, kefir, ricotta, farmer cheese, yogurt). If you use SWAMI personalized nutrition report, there could be cheeses that are more or less *Beneficial* than others, so focus on those.
Eggs
Poultry (chicken, Cornish hen, turkey)

Filling up Your Freezer
Smoothies

Making smoothies is a great alternative for breakfast or a delicious, protein-filled snack. When fruit is in season, fresh fruit can be used, however, mix some frozen fruits and vegetables into the smoothie for a thicker consistency.

BENEFICIALS

Apricots	Figs
Blackberries	Kale
Blueberries	Pineapple
Cherries	Spinach

NEUTRALS

Avocado	Peaches	Strawberries
Dates	Raspberries	

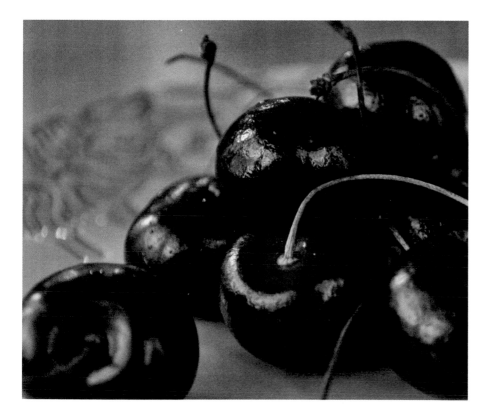

Leftovers

It's always helpful to double the recipe when making foods that freeze easily such as:

Chili	Lasagna	Sauces
Cookies	Muffins	Stew
Crackers	Pesto	

Pesto can be stored in BPA-free ice cube trays for individual servings. In the following pages you will find more information on safe food storage as well as suggestions for cooking in bulk.

Protein

It is helpful for weeknight dinners to keep at least a few protein options in the freezer. To defrost poultry or seafood, take them out the day before and put them in the refrigerator.

BENEFICIALS
Turkey (ground turkey, tenderloins)
Seafood (carp, cod, mackerel, monkfish, perch, pickerel, pollack, red snapper, salmon, sardine, snail, trout, whitefish, whiting)

Time to Get in That Pantry
Snacks

The first thing we all go into the pantry for is to grab a quick bite on the run or pack a snack to ship off to school with the kids. It is important that these midday treats are balanced and wholesome, especially to keep your blood sugar balanced, so the best way to make that happen is to stock that pantry right. Here are a few staples for Type A:

BENEFICIALS
Brown rice cakes
Dark chocolate (70 percent or higher)
Dried fruit (apricots, cherries, figs, prunes)
Flaxseeds
Fresh fruit (pineapple, blueberries, cherries, grapefruit, plums)
Nuts (walnuts, peanuts, almonds, pecans, macadamias)

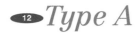

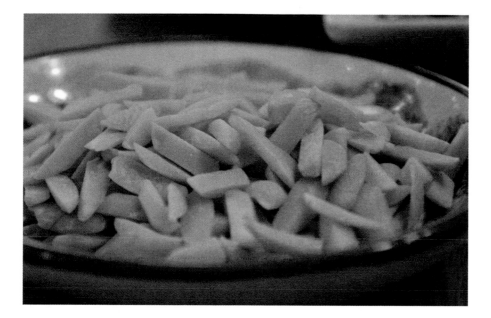

Peanut butter
Pumpkin seeds

If you want to prep ahead for those times when you are in a rush, make individual servings of combinations of nuts, dried fruit, and maybe even a little dark chocolate. Store in small, glass, sealable containers and take them in the car, on the plane, or anywhere you are headed.

Bread

As a Type A, you are among the few who can tolerate wheat. That being said, it is a *Neutral*, so if you want to focus on grains that are *Beneficial* to your diet, opt for Ezekiel breads (made from sprouted wheat) or breads made of oat or rye flour. Please note that the commercial version of Ezekiel bread now adds wheat gluten, so be sure to check ingredient lists for potential *Avoid* foods added.

Drinks

Yet another reason you are lucky to be Type A: coffee and red wine are actually highly *Beneficial* for you. Of course it's not advisable to drink either of them throughout the day, so aside from water, when you want to add a little flavor to your beverage repertoire, dabble in these *Beneficial* teas or fruit juices, plain or with a touch of lemon/lime or mint. In fact, as a Type A, it is a good idea to start the day with warm water with a squeeze of lemon. A few recipes for teas can be found in this book.

BENEFICIALS
Aloe juice
Coffee
Fruit juice (black cherry)
Red wine
Teas (chamomile, dandelion, echinacea, green, ginger, ginseng, chamomile, ginseng, rose hip)

Grains/Legumes

Whole grains and legumes are *Beneficial* to your diet, so try to incorporate them when you can. Always keep these ingredients on hand so they are readily available for your use.

BENEFICIALS
Beans (adzuki, black, black-eyed peas, fava, lentils, soybeans, pinto)
Whole grains (buckwheat, oat flour, oatmeal, rye flour)

NEUTRALS
Whole grains (barley, corn, couscous, millet, quinoa, rice, wheat, spelt)

Seasonings

Making healthy food taste good is non-negotiable. One quick trick is knowing your way around your spice cabinet. Herbs and spices are calorie free and flavor packed. The spices listed below also happen to be terrific for your Type A body. Keep a jar of homemade Basic Bread Crumbs on hand for a quick topping on a casserole, to use as turkey breading or to bread seafood. Olive oil is also a good thing to keep on hand. Additionally, as much as we would like to repress our sweet tooth, it is an unrealistic expectation for most, so stock up on natural sweeteners like agave and maple syrup, but use sparingly.

BENEFICIALS
Agave nectar
Basic Bread Crumbs NS (page 210)
Blackstrap molasses

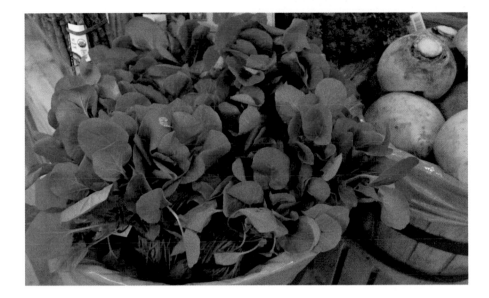

Honey
Maple syrup
Miso
Olive oil
Soy sauce
Vanilla
Spices (garlic, ginger, horseradish, mustard, tamari)

NEUTRALS
  Spices (allspice, basil, bay leaf, caraway, cardamom, chives, cinnamon,
     clove, coriander, nutmeg, oregano, paprika, peppermint, saffron,
     rosemary, sage, tarragon, thyme, sea salt)

Recipe Ideas for Last-Minute Cooking

Time-Saving Tricks

Make these recipes in bulk and store in your freezer to grab on the go: Flax
chips, smoothies in individual portions, baked goods, granola, soups, casseroles, sauces, pesto in ice-cube trays, and stews.

When making dressings or condiments, double or triple the recipe and
store it in the refrigerator for future use. If you are making the recipe with
one lemon, you might as well do it with three and save yourself the prep
and clean-up again and again.

 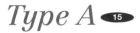

Utilize Roasted Vegetables

Let's reemphasize here how amazingly useful leftover roasted vegetables can be. Not only are they ready to be thrown into just about any dish, but they add tremendous flavor with no effort whatsoever. Here are a few examples where you can toss in roasted vegetables and have a tasty new dish:

Casseroles	Omelets	Soufflés
Cold pasta salad	Pizza	Spring rolls
Crêpes	Quiches	Tacos
Frittata	Rice salads	Vegetable tarts
Lettuce wraps	Salads	

Next time you make roasted vegetables for dinner, do yourself a favor and double up on that recipe.

Review Your Stock

Now that you have the basics, it's time to take a look at some of the *Avoids*. You have lived your whole life eating whatever you want. Now you open your cabinets and think, how do I start over?, but the answer is simple: you don't have to. You just have to emphasize the healthy choices that you are now privy to. You should ditch anything that is categorized *Best Avoided* for your type; listed below are a few places where *Avoids* may be lurking and ready to sabotage your otherwise perfect, new diet.

- Open up the fridge—take inventory of all condiments, sauces, stocks, and other processed foods.
- Open the pantry—familiarize yourself with ingredients in your snacks, cereals, pastas, spices, and other foods.
- Open the freezer—remove frozen dinners. Just do it. You can be sure they are not doing you any good. Other than that, the same applies here as above: evaluate what you have, and review ingredients just to get yourself acquainted with what you are dealing with.

Once you have done that, take out all questionable foods and line them up on the counter or table. Refer to your Type A diet in the book *Eat Right For Your Type*, or you can use Type Base Food Values online (www .dadamo.com). If you do have a personalized plan, refer to your SWAMI

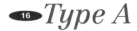

reference book. Check out your *Avoids*, as this will be the most efficient way of eliminating those foods that are best *Avoided*.

Here is a rundown of some of the main offenders:

Meat

The very first thing Type As notice and either become excited about or cringe over is that it is best to give up beef. Unless you have a very acute illness that requires immediate, strict adherence to the diet, it is okay to ease into this. Take your time and focus on the foods that are *Beneficial* to you and try to eat them as often as possible. If giving up meat is difficult to envision, understand the 80/20 rule . . . unless you are acutely ill, eating right for your blood type 80 percent of the time will give you full results. The last thing we want is for you to stress out, or not start the diet over eliminating meat.

Vinegar

You are a Type A, and vinegar is an *Avoid* for you. I know you might be cringing at the thought of living sans vinegar—I know I was. But don't fret; I will give you recipes to fill the void. For now, let's get it out of your kitchen—out of sight, out of mind. So, the big question is, where does vinegar lurk when the word *vinegar* is not in the name—as in balsamic, red wine, apple cider, or rice wine vinegars?

The following foods can contain vinegar:

Chili sauces	Prepared horseradish
Cocktail sauce	Prepared mustard
Ketchup	Relishes
Mayonnaise	Salad dressings
Olives	Steak sauce
Pickles	Worcestershire sauce
Pickled vegetables	

Peppers (Spice)

Although most vegetables are healing for your body, peppers are not among them. There are many varieties of peppers, from sweet bell peppers to spicy chipotle, so this is just a little reminder to be wary of anything spicy. The only exceptions to pepper in your diet are two *Neutrals*: paprika and pimiento pepper. You will see them both in the recipes in this book; they are acceptable for your type.

The Rest

Other than meat, vinegar, and peppers, it will be straightforward to determine what to take out of your cabinets, fridge, and freezer. Take the time to go through your list of *Avoids* and remove them from your house. If you have canned goods and non-perishables, you can donate to your local food bank. To find a food bank in your area, go to: http://feeding america.org. Again, unless you are acutely sick and can apply the 80/20 rule to save money you can phase out the *Avoids* by only eating them once in a while until they are gone and then filling your cabinets with only *Neutrals* and *Beneficials*.

You should be all cleared out, so now you are ready to go to the store and grab a few essentials to fill in the gaps.

How to Read These Recipes

This cookbook for the blood Type A individual is designed to be as practical and helpful to the Blood Type dieter as possible. We took into consideration that many families could be cooking for multiple blood types or preparing meals for friends with varying blood types. In order to make doing so practical, each of the *Eat Right 4 Your Type* cookbooks contains the same or similar recipe ideas with different executions to suit the needs of each blood type. You will find the recipe titles almost identical in each book; however, ingredients and methods might vary quite a bit. There are many recipes that are *Beneficial* across the board and are marked with a (A/B/AB/O) to identify that they are universal to every type. For example, every blood type has a pancake recipe; however, the Type A recipe has *Beneficial* grains that might be on the *Avoid* list for other types, so each recipe contains different flours. Every recipe is also written to contain as many *Beneficial* foods as possible, while understanding that taste is still of the utmost importance. After all, you are not going to be inclined to dive into a kale cookie, but you won't be able to resist Pasta Carbonara with Crispy Kale. The point is that we want you coming back for more each time to see that eating right for your blood type is as far from sacrifice as is indulging in a bar of chocolate.

As you make your way through this book, you will notice that once in a while there is a highlighted section called "Featured Ingredient." There are several ingredients used in this book that you may not have come across before, some that are *Beneficial* for your diet and some that are *Beneficial* for your taste buds. In an effort to familiarize you with these ingredients, there is a brief summary explaining a little about what that ingredient is, and how or why it is used. Don't be afraid to experiment with unfamiliar territory; let this book be your guide as you open new culinary doors.

Many people who follow the Blood Type Diet have seen me or used the tests on my website (www. 4yourtype.com) to create a specific diet plan for each individual. If you have done that, you have a SWAMI personalized nutrition report that may vary slightly from the general Type A diet because it takes into consideration family and medical history, Secretor Status, and GenoType. (The GenoType is a further refinement of my work in personalized nutrition. It uses a variety of simple measurements, combined with blood type status to classify individuals as one of six basic Epigenotypes: the Hunter, Gatherer, Teacher, Explorer, Warrior, and Nomad types.) Due to the variations in *Beneficial*, *Neutral*, and *Best Avoided* foods, there may be some recipes containing ingredients that do not suit you as an individual. Please do not skip these recipes entirely. There is always a way to make quick and easy substitutions. (See "Useful Tools: Substitutions," page 213.) As a quick piece of advice, vegetables can be easily swapped out—leafy greens for other leafy greens, a specific type of beans for another or in some cases, simply omitted from the recipe if it is not a star component.

You will see that recipes are also tagged according to Secretor Status. Some recipes are not appropriate for Non-Secretors but are fine for Secretors (see the recipe legend on the following page). In most instances when this is the case, there are simple substitutions to adapt the recipe for Non-Secretors. In a few cases, however, the recipe will be an *Avoid* altogether for a Type A Non-Secretor.

In many of the recipes in this book, you will see sea salt written as "sea salt, to taste" and might be wondering what that means or how much to add. Salt can make or break your dish; if you add too much, there is no going back. Add a little at a time; taste and add more if needed. What is *a little*? Well, start with pinching a bit between your fingers and sprinkling it into your dish, give it a minute to incorporate, and then taste. If you were to measure a pinch, it would be a little less than ⅛ teaspoon.

As you know at this point, one of the major changes for most people following the Type A diet is becoming meat-free. Throughout the book, recipes that could use meat as a star ingredient are replaced with tofu, tempeh, or some kind of poultry. If you have the reaction to the idea of tofu or tempeh that most people do the first time they see it, this may be a very unappealing swap for you. The best part about tofu is that it is a blank canvas for any of your favorite flavor combinations. When marinated in soy, honey, and ginger, for example, and then seared in a bit of olive oil, tofu is transformed into a delicious and desirable meal, one you will certainly not shun the next time around.

Remember to read each recipe in its entirety before making it to ensure you know how much time it will take and if there are any ingredients you will need to buy ahead of time. Finally, enjoy making, eating, and sharing these recipes.

RECIPE LEGEND:

- An * is used when a recipe ingredient needs further instruction, substitution, or comment. This information is found at the bottom of a recipe.
- All recipes are appropriate for Type A Secretors.
- (NS) represents a recipe that is appropriate for Type A Non-Secretors.
- Recipe ingredients that are NOT appropriate for Type A Non-Secretors (NS) are notated with appropriate acceptable substitutions within recipe ingredients.

A REVIEW OF THE FOOD LISTS

Throughout this book we refer to a number of places to find the comprehensive foods lists for the Blood Type Diet. Here's a recap of where you can find the lists so you can use the one that is right for you:

- *Eat Right 4 Your Type*, which provides the entry point into the Blood Type Diet
- *Live Right 4 Your Type*, which incorporates the value of the Secretor Status
- *Blood Type A Food, Beverage, and Supplement Lists from Eat Right 4 Your Type*, a handy pocket guide with the basic food lists
- *Change Your Genetic Destiny* (originally published as *The Geno-Type Diet*, which provides a further refinement of the diet by using blood type, secretor status, and a series of biometric measurements to further individualize your food lists)
- SWAMI Personalized Nutrition Software. Designed to harness the power of computers and artificial intelligence, using their tremendous precision and speed to help tailor unique, one-of-a-kind diets. From its extensive knowledge base, SWAMI can evaluate more than 700 foods for more than 200 individual attributes (such as cholesterol level, gluten content, presence of antioxidants, etc.) to determine if that food is either a superfood or toxin for you. It provides a specific, unique diet in an easy-to-read, user-friendly format, complete with food lists, recipes, and meal planning.

Breakfast

Breakfast recipes were written with diversity in mind, so that you do not end up eating the same thing every day. The idea here is to alternate: one day eggs, the next quinoa or granola, and so on, in order to keep providing your body with different nutrients each day. You will probably notice the biggest changes in these recipes are the types of flour used. Don't be intimidated; try one simple recipe like the pancakes to get your feet wet and move on to the rest. Once you have the new flour on hand, the rest is just like any other recipe.

Quinoa Muesli 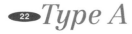NS

½ cup quinoa

½ cup water

½ cup almond milk plus more if needed

¼ teaspoon sea salt

2 tablespoons dried cherries

1 tablespoon dried cranberries

2 tablespoons slivered almonds

2 tablespoons chopped walnuts

¼ teaspoon cinnamon

2 teaspoons maple syrup

¼ cup crunchy rice cereal

1. Rinse quinoa. In a small saucepan, add quinoa, water, almond milk, sea salt, cherries, and cranberries, and bring to a boil. Cook 10 minutes, turn off the heat, and let sit an additional 4 to 5 minutes. Quinoa will absorb all the water and become light and fluffy when done.

2. While the quinoa cooks, toast almonds and walnuts in a dry skillet over medium heat for about 2 minutes or until slightly golden brown. Watch nuts carefully; they have a tendency to burn easily because of their high fat content.

3. Fluff cooked quinoa with a fork, and add toasted nuts, cinnamon, and maple syrup. Top with crunchy rice cereal, and add more almond milk, if desired.

4. Serve immediately.

▶ SERVES 2

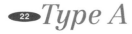

EAT RIGHT FOR YOUR TYPE PERSONALIZED COOKBOOK

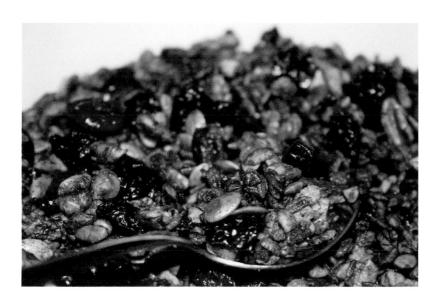

Blackstrap-Cherry Granola NS

4 cups crispy rice cereal

1 cup chopped walnuts

1 cup chopped pecans

¼ cup whole flaxseeds

¼ cup blackstrap molasses

2 teaspoons olive oil

1 tablespoon agave

⅛ teaspoon sea salt

¼ cup water

1 cup halved dried cherries

½ cup halved dried cranberries

1. Preheat oven to 350 degrees. Line a sheet pan with parchment paper and set aside.

2. In a large bowl, combine rice cereal, walnuts, pecans, and flaxseeds, and set aside.

3. In a small saucepan, warm molasses, olive oil, agave, and salt with water over medium heat for about 2 minutes, whisking to combine.

4. Pour the liquid over granola mixture, toss to coat, and spread onto prepared pan. Bake 10 minutes.

5. Take granola out of the oven. Toss, and place back in the oven, reducing the temperature to 300 degrees.

6. Bake an additional 25 minutes.

7. Toss granola with cherries and cranberries.

8. Serve warm or cool fully, and store in an airtight, glass container for up to 2 weeks or in the freezer for up to 2 months.

▶ YIELDS 32 (¼ CUP) SERVINGS

 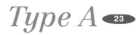

Granola–Nut Butter Fruit Slices NS

3 tablespoons peanut butter

⅓ cup granola*

¼ teaspoon cinnamon

Sea salt, to taste

1 pear

1 apple

1 lemon

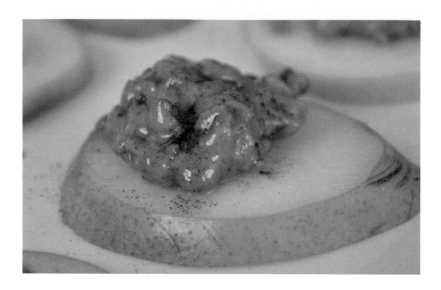

1. Combine peanut butter, granola, and cinnamon, until granola is evenly coated. Season with sea salt to taste.

2. Thinly slice pear and apple into ¼-inch rounds. Cut lemon in half and rub cut side on fruit pieces to prevent browning. Spoon 1 to 2 teaspoons of the granola mixture on fruit and enjoy!

*See Blackstrap-Cherry Granola NS recipe (page 23).

▶ SERVES 4

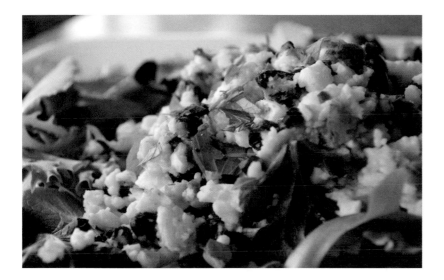

Breakfast Egg Salad NS

dressing:

½ teaspoon mustard powder

1 tablespoon olive oil

1 tablespoon lemon juice

1 tablespoon onion, grated

Sea salt, to taste

2 teaspoons olive oil

½ cup cooked or canned black-eyed peas, drained and rinsed

3 large hard-boiled eggs

¼ cup grated mozzarella cheese

1 tablespoon chopped parsley

2 cups mixed baby greens

Sea salt, to taste

1. Whisk together all dressing ingredients, and set aside.

2. In a small skillet, heat olive oil over medium heat. Toast black-eyed peas for 2 to 3 minutes until warm and slightly crunchy. Set aside.

3. Remove eggs from shells, and use a fork to break apart in a bowl. Add beans, cheese, and parsley to eggs, and toss with dressing. Season with sea salt, to taste. Serve over mixed baby greens.

▶ SERVES 4

Type A 25

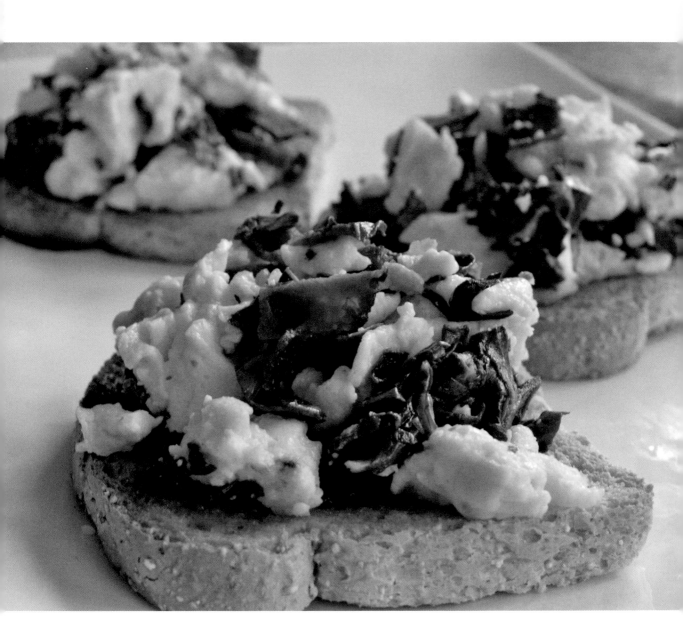

Nonstick cooking spray
3 strips turkey bacon
3 large eggs
3 large egg whites
2 teaspoons olive oil
2 cups fresh spinach
Sea salt, to taste
¼ cup mozzarella cheese
4 slices Ezekiel bread, toasted

1. Heat a large skillet over medium heat and coat with nonstick cooking spray.

2. Once the skillet is hot, add bacon and let cook 3 to 4 minutes, flip, and cook an additional 2 to 3 minutes on the opposite side for crispy bacon.* Remove from pan, let cool, crumble, and set aside.

3. Whisk eggs and egg whites in a small bowl. In the same skillet as the bacon, add olive oil and reduce heat slightly. Add spinach and sauté 2 minutes, season mixture with sea salt. Pour eggs over spinach, cooking gently until done, about 2 additional minutes. Turn off heat and add reserved bacon and cheese.

4. Spoon mixture on toast and serve immediately.

*If the bacon is not as crispy as you like, you can add a drizzle of olive oil to help it along.

▶ SERVES 4

featured ingredient

turkey bacon (nitrate-/preservative-free)

Not all turkey bacon is the same. There are many types/brands on the market, but most are artificially derived, loaded with salt and preservatives, and full of nitrates . . . all things you absolutely do not want to be eating. There are a few companies that make turkey bacon without these unhealthy and artificial additives; they can be found at your local natural food store and in some mainstream grocery stores.

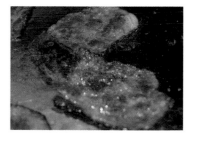

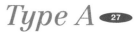

Swiss Chard and Cremini Frittata NS

2 teaspoons ghee

¼ cup finely diced Spanish onion

1 cup diced cremini mushrooms*

3 cups chopped Swiss chard

3 large egg whites

3 large eggs

2 tablespoons spelt flour

Sea salt, to taste

1 teaspoon chopped fresh tarragon

1 teaspoon olive oil

1 tablespoon pepitas (sunflower seeds), toasted

1. Preheat oven to 375 degrees.

2. In a sauté pan, heat ghee over medium heat. Sauté onion, mushrooms, and Swiss chard for 4 to 5 minutes, until vegetables become tender.

3. While onion mixture is cooking, whisk together eggs, egg whites, flour, salt, and tarragon. Add olive oil to skillet, and pour egg mixture over vegetables. Cook for 1 minute.

4. Transfer to oven and bake for 6 to 8 minutes, or until firm and edges are golden. Top with pepitas and serve warm.

*Note: Cremini mushrooms are also known as baby portabella mushrooms.

▶ SERVES 4

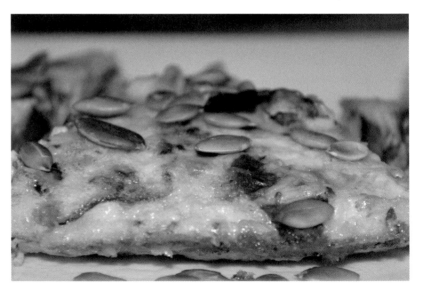

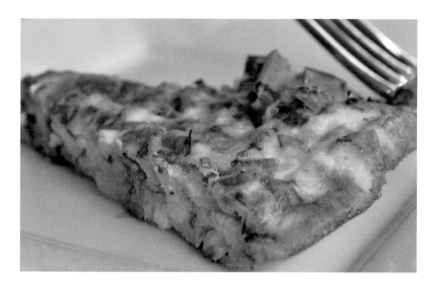

Broccoli-Feta Frittata 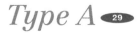 NS

1 head broccoli

¼ teaspoon sea salt

1 tablespoon plus 2 teaspoons olive oil

3 large eggs

2 large egg whites

⅓ cup crumbled feta

½ cup chopped spinach

¼ cup finely diced chives

2 teaspoons spelt flour

1 tablespoon chopped oregano

1. Preheat oven to 375 degrees.

2. Dice broccoli into bite-size pieces and place in single layer on a baking sheet. Sprinkle with a dash of sea salt and 1 tablespoon olive oil. Bake 15 minutes. Set aside.

3. In a medium-size bowl, whisk eggs, egg whites, feta, spinach, chives, flour, oregano, and additional salt to taste until well combined.

4. Brush remaining 2 teaspoons olive oil across a medium-size skillet over medium heat, to create a nonstick surface. Once warm, add egg mixture and broccoli. Cook 1 to 2 minutes, lifting the side of the eggs gently with your spatula to encourage uncooked egg to run down into the bottom of the skillet.

5. Place skillet under the broiler for 2 minutes, or until the eggs set and brown very slightly on the edges. If the handle of your skillet is rubber, wrap tightly with tinfoil to prevent melting.

6. Serve warm.

▶ SERVES 4

Type A 29

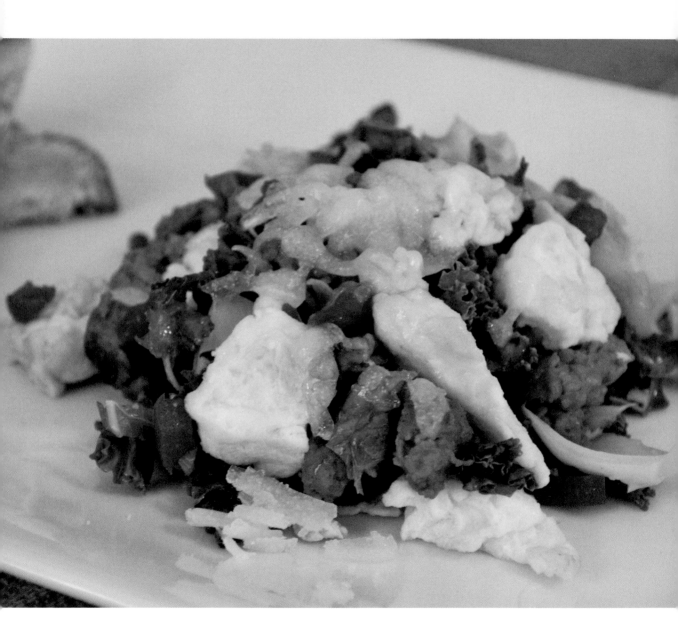

Maple-Sausage Scramble (NS)

1. In large skillet, sauté onion, kale, and artichokes in 2 teaspoons olive oil over medium heat for 3 to 4 minutes. Remove veggies from skillet and set aside. Brown turkey sausage in the same skillet with remaining olive oil, breaking up sausage into bite-size pieces until cooked through, about 5 to 6 minutes. Drizzle with maple syrup and stir to distribute over sausage. Add to veggies and set aside.

2. Whisk eggs and egg whites with water and salt, and add to skillet, reducing the heat to medium-low. Stir gently with a heat-safe spatula until firm and cooked through. Return sausage and veggie mixture to the skillet with the eggs and stir to combine.

3. Serve topped with shredded cheese.

▶ **SERVES 4**

¼ cup finely chopped white onion

3 cups chopped kale

2 cups frozen artichoke hearts, thawed and quartered

1 tablespoon olive oil, divided

½ pound raw turkey sausage

1 tablespoon maple syrup

3 large eggs

2 large egg whites

1 tablespoon water

Sea salt, to taste

¼ cup shredded mozzarella cheese

Homemade Turkey Breakfast Sausage

2 teaspoons olive oil

½ cup finely diced onion

½ cup finely diced fennel

1 pound ground turkey meat

1 teaspoon fennel seed

1 teaspoon paprika

1 teaspoon sea salt

1 clove garlic, minced

½ cup finely diced Bosc pear

2 teaspoons maple syrup

1. In a large sauté pan, heat olive oil over medium heat and add onions and fennel. Sauté 3 to 4 minutes or until tender. Remove from heat and let cool to room temperature, about 10 minutes.

2. Once the vegetables are cool, place ground turkey in a large bowl, and add fennel seed, paprika, salt, garlic, pear, maple syrup, and cooled vegetables. Use your hands to incorporate all ingredients into the meat, but do not over mix.

3. Form meat into small, hot dog–shaped logs. Cook 8 to 10 minutes or until meat is browned on all sides and inside of the sausage is no longer pink.

4. Serve warm alone or alongside scrambled eggs for a protein-packed breakfast!

▶ SERVES 4

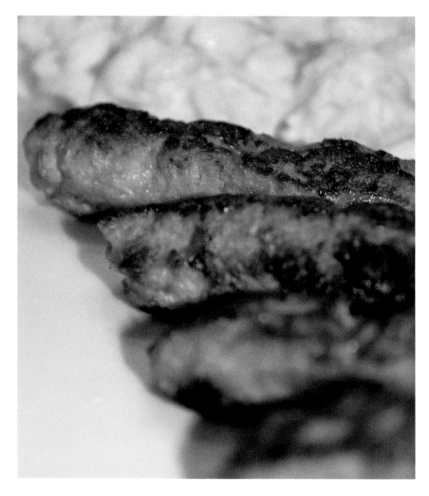

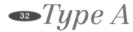

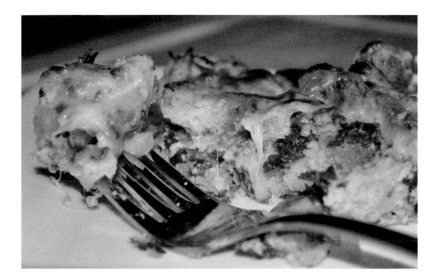

Savory Herb and Cheese Bread Pudding NS

1. Preheat oven to 350 degrees. Grease a 9" x 11" baking dish with nonstick cooking spray (olive oil from a refillable oil mister would work well) and set aside.

2. In a large skillet, heat olive oil and ghee over medium heat. Sauté onions, mushrooms, zucchini, and kale until tender, about 5 to 6 minutes. Season with salt and set aside.

3. Spread bread cubes in a single layer on a baking sheet. Toast for 3 to 4 minutes until slightly golden brown. Toss in a large bowl with vegetables.

4. Whisk together almond milk, stock, eggs, rosemary, sage, and thyme. Pour over bread and vegetables and toss. Pour the entire mixture onto the baking dish. Top with mozzarella cheese and bake, covered for 35 minutes. Remove the cover and bake an additional 10 minutes, until cheese is bubbling and slightly browned.

5. Serve warm.

*See Vegetable Stock NS recipe (page 210).

▶ SERVES 12

Nonstick cooking spray

2 cups diced onion

2 cups quartered cremini mushrooms

2 cups diced zucchini

6 cups torn kale

2 teaspoons olive oil

1 teaspoon ghee

Sea salt, to taste

8 cups (1-inch) bread cubes (sprouted wheat or spelt)

1 cup almond milk

1 cup Vegetable Stock*

4 large eggs, beaten

1 teaspoon finely chopped fresh rosemary

1 teaspoon finely chopped fresh sage

1 teaspoon fresh thyme

1 cup mozzarella cheese

Spinach and Zucchini Soufflé 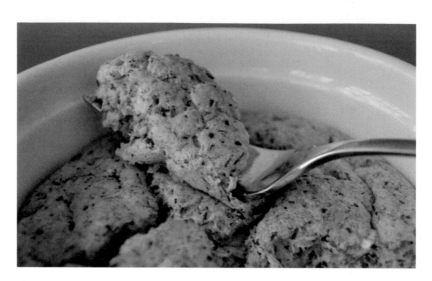 NS

Nonstick cooking spray
1 tablespoon ghee
2 tablespoons oat flour
½ cup soy or almond milk
½ cup Vegetable Stock*
2 cups packed spinach
2 cups chopped zucchini
2 large egg yolks
¼ cup chopped basil
¼ cup crumbled feta cheese
⅛ teaspoon ground cloves
4 large egg whites, at room temperature

1. Preheat oven to 350 degrees. Spray 4 (12-oz.) ramekins with nonstick cooking spray and set aside.

2. In a saucepan over medium heat, melt ghee and whisk in flour. Gradually add soy milk and stock, whisking continuously until thickened, about 3 to 4 minutes. Once mixture is thick and resembles the consistency of yogurt, remove from the heat and cool completely.

3. In a food processor, puree spinach and zucchini; strain excess liquid through cheesecloth or paper towels. Place vegetables in a bowl and whisk in egg yolks, basil, cheese, and cloves. Set aside.

4. Once cooled, fold milk mixture into vegetable mixture.

5. In a dry, glass bowl, beat egg whites with a hand mixer until they form stiff peaks. Fold the egg whites, one-third at a time, into the vegetables. Spoon mixture into prepared ramekins, and set on a baking dish. Fill baking dish halfway with hot water. Carefully place in the oven and bake for 45 minutes or until tester comes out clean.

6. Serve immediately.

*See Vegetable Stock NS recipe (page 210).

▶ SERVES 4

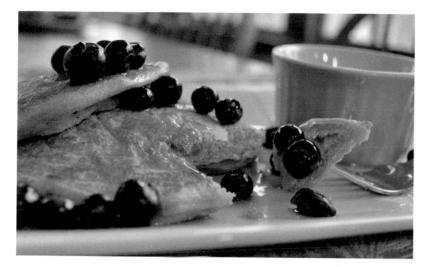

Pancakes NS

¾ cup spelt flour

¼ cup oat flour

2 teaspoons baking powder

½ teaspoon sea salt

2 large eggs

1 cup almond or soy milk

2 tablespoons olive oil

Nonstick cooking spray

1. In a large bowl, combine flours, baking powder, and salt. Set aside.

2. In a separate bowl, whisk eggs, milk, and olive oil. Add to flour mixture, and stir until well combined and free of lumps.

3. Spray a skillet with nonstick cooking spray and place over medium heat. Spoon ¼ cup batter into skillet, and let cook 1 to 2 minutes per side.

4. Serve warm.

▶ SERVES 4

tip: If making a large batch, keep warm in the oven at 200 degrees, draped with a slightly damp paper towel.

featured ingredient

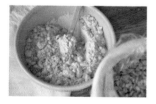

oat flour

Oats have a delicious, creamy flavor and add smooth texture to baked goods. You can make oat flour yourself by grinding quick-cooking oats in your food processor until fine. Naturally rich in fiber, one benefit of including oats in your diet is their ability to satiate your appetite, so you will not feel hungry soon after your meal. Oat flour is not self-rising because it does not contain gluten, so it's best to combine it with spelt or wheat when baking. This is why most of the recipes in this book call for a combination of oat and spelt flours.

 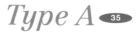

Cinnamon-Oat Crêpes NS

⅔ cup oat flour

⅓ cup spelt flour

¼ teaspoon sea salt

¼ teaspoon cinnamon

1¼ cups soy or goat milk

2 large eggs

1 tablespoon plus 1 teaspoon melted ghee, divided

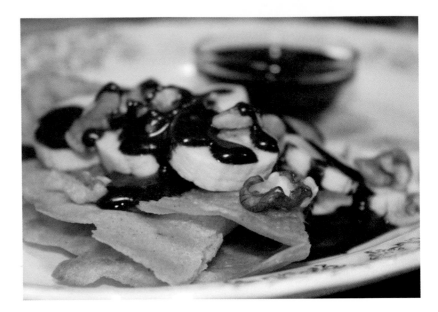

1. In a medium bowl, whisk flours, sea salt, and cinnamon. Set aside.

2. Beat milk, eggs, and 1 tablespoon ghee. Add to flour mixture, and whisk until well blended. Cover and let sit 1 hour.

3. Heat a large sauté pan over medium heat. When the pan is hot, add remaining 1 teaspoon ghee and brush evenly across the bottom of the pan. Use a ¼-cup measuring cup to scoop batter, pour into pan and quickly turn the pan in circular motions to spread the batter into a very thin layer. Let cook 1 minute or until the batter firms, and edges lift slightly off the pan. Use an offset spatula to flip, and cook another minute.

▶ SERVES 4

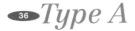

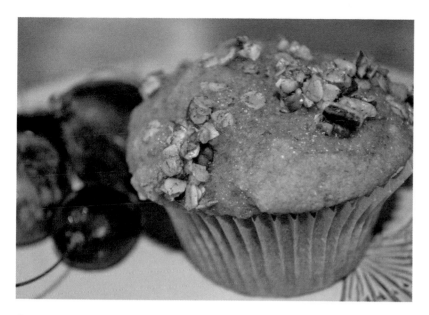

Pumpkin Muffins with Carob Drizzle (NS)

1. Preheat oven to 350 degrees. Line a 12-cup muffin pan with paper liners and set aside.

2. In a large bowl, stir flours, baking powder, baking soda, salt, cinnamon, cloves, ginger, and allspice until well combined.

3. In a separate bowl, whisk pumpkin, honey, eggs, and milk. Add the pumpkin mixture to the flour mixture and stir to incorporate. Spoon into prepared muffin tins.

4. Combine oats, pecans, cinnamon, honey, and oil in a small bowl and toss with a fork. Sprinkle topping evenly on each muffin and drizzle with Carob Extract.

5. Bake 20 to 25 minutes or until a toothpick inserted into muffins comes out clean.

*Information about purchasing Carob Extract™ can be found in Appendix II: Products (page 233).

▶ SERVES 12

2 cups spelt flour

1 cup oat flour

2 teaspoons baking powder

½ teaspoon baking soda

½ teaspoon fine sea salt

1 teaspoon ground cinnamon

⅛ teaspoon ground cloves

½ teaspoon ground ginger

¼ teaspoon allspice

1 (15-oz.) can organic pumpkin puree

½ cup honey

2 large eggs

½ cup soy milk

topping:

¼ cup rolled oats

⅓ cup finely chopped pecans

½ teaspoon ground cinnamon

1 tablespoon honey

1 tablespoon walnut or light olive oil

¼ cup Carob Extract*

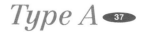

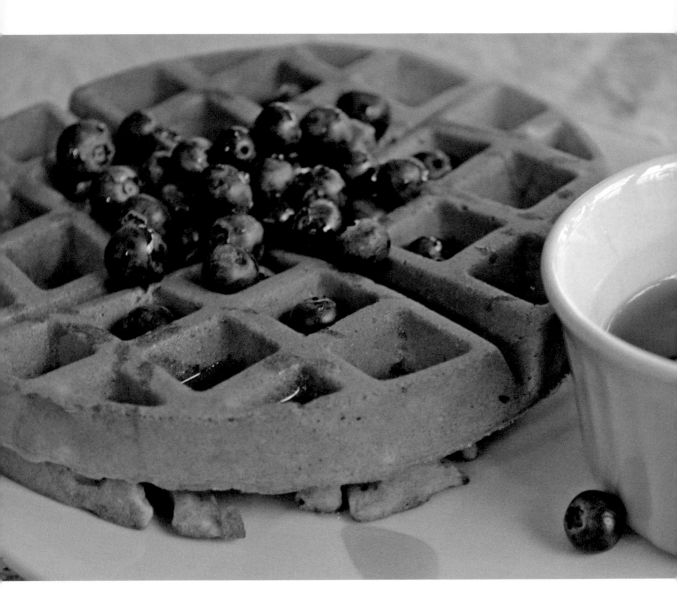

Wild-Rice Waffles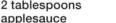

1. Preheat waffle maker.

2. In a large bowl, whisk dry ingredients until well combined.

3. In a separate bowl, whisk eggs, milk, olive oil, and applesauce. Add wet ingredients to dry and mix until free of lumps. Fold in cooked rice.

4. Spoon batter into waffle maker filled just to the rims, close, and cook according to settings on your waffle maker. Waffles should be firm with a slightly crunchy exterior and soft interior.

5. Serve warm.

▶ SERVES 4

1½ cups spelt flour

½ cup oat flour

2 tablespoons flaxseeds

½ teaspoon sea salt

2 teaspoons baking powder

¼ teaspoon cinnamon

2 large eggs

2 cups soy or goat milk

2 tablespoons olive oil

2 tablespoons applesauce

1 cup cooked wild rice

featured ingredient

flaxseeds

Flaxseeds are small with a hard, smooth surface and are packed with omega-3 fatty acids as well as manganese, fiber, and other nutrients. Foods rich in omega-3s are a healthy addition to any diet and provide anti-inflammatory benefits for Type As, specifically in their ability to fight cancer and diabetes. Flaxseeds can be added to smoothies, baked goods, or even used as a topping on salads. When submerged in warm water, flaxseeds bind together with the water and form a gelatin that is helpful in gluten-free baking, and if drunk will help keep you "regular."

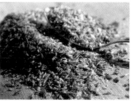

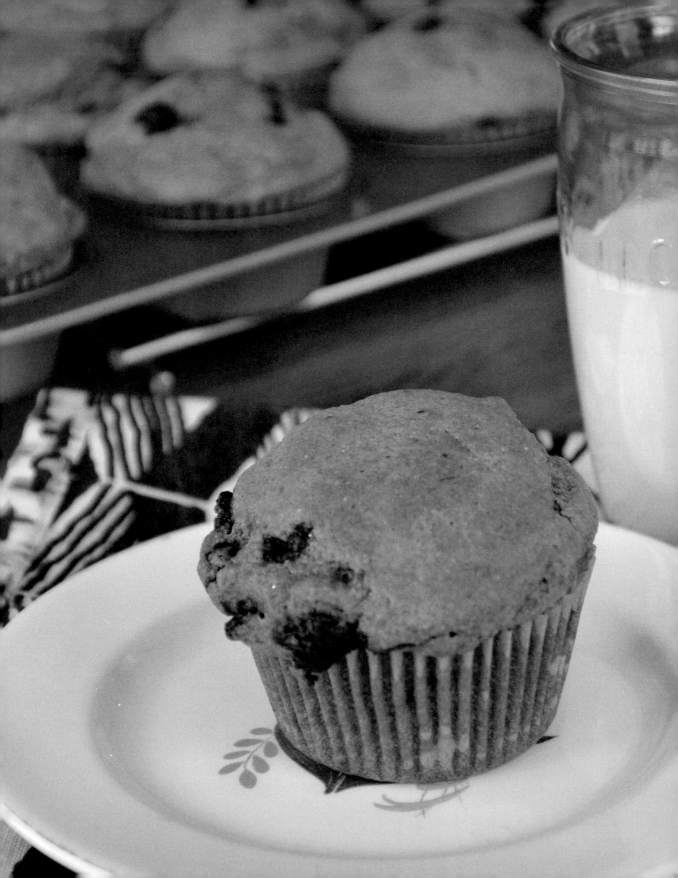

Blueberry-Macadamia Muffins NS

1. Preheat oven to 350 degrees. Line a 12-cup muffin pan with paper liners and set aside.

2. In a large bowl, combine dry ingredients. Set aside.

3. In a separate bowl, whisk wet ingredients.

4. Add the wet ingredients to the dry, stirring to combine. Fold in macadamia nuts and blueberries. Spoon batter evenly into prepared muffin tins, and bake for 25 to 28 minutes, or until toothpick inserted into muffins comes out clean.

▶ SERVES 12

1½ cups spelt flour

1 cup oat flour

½ teaspoon salt

2 teaspoons baking powder

1 teaspoon baking soda

½ teaspoon cinnamon

2 large eggs

½ cup agave

½ teaspoon lemon zest

3 tablespoons light olive oil

½ cup applesauce

½ cup plus 2 tablespoons soy or almond milk

½ cup chopped macadamia nuts

1 cup (fresh or frozen) organic blueberries

featured ingredient

almond milk

As the name indicates, almond milk is, in fact, made from ground almonds processed with water. It is low in calories, contains no cholesterol or lactose, and has a slightly sweet, creamy flavor that is a perfect replacement to cow milk. It can be used as a direct replacement for cow milk in most recipes, including baked goods, beverages, and some sauces. Interestingly, almond milk was quite popular in the Middle Ages due to its high protein content and prolonged shelf life.

Cherry Scones (NS)

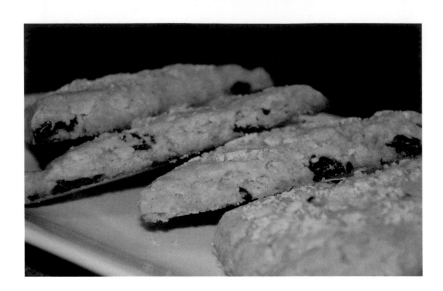

scones:

½ cup dried cherries, halved

1 cup spelt flour, plus more for rolling

½ cup oat flour

¼ cup almond flour

2 teaspoons baking powder

½ teaspoon sea salt

4 tablespoons cold unsalted butter

¼ cup almond milk

1 large egg

1 teaspoon lemon zest

⅓ cup agave

topping:

2 tablespoons agave

2 tablespoons almond flour

1. Preheat oven to 350 degrees. Line a baking sheet with parchment paper and set aside.

2. Place dried cherries in a small bowl and rehydrate them by covering with steaming-hot water for 10 minutes. Remove, pat dry, and set aside.

3. In a large mixing bowl, combine flours with baking powder and salt. Stir to combine.

4. Cut cold butter into small cubes and cut into the flour mixture using a pastry cutter or two butter knives. Continue until flour resembles coarse corn meal. Toss cherries into dry mixture, making sure they are evenly distributed throughout the flour.

5. In a separate bowl, whisk milk, egg, lemon zest, and agave until well combined. Fold the milk mixture into the dry mixture until well combined. Dough will be thick and slightly sticky. Use extra flour to form the dough into a ball. Gently place on a floured surface and use your hands to pat the dough into a rectangular shape about 1 inch thick. Using a sharp knife, cut the dough horizontally once and then into thirds vertically, to make 6 squares. Cut each square again at an angle to make 12 triangles. Gently place each scone onto prepared baking sheet. Brush the tops evenly with agave and then sprinkle with almond flour.

6. Bake 20 to 22 minutes or until firm and lightly browned on the bottoms. Serve warm or let cool completely and store in a cool, dry place overnight.

7. Scones can be frozen for up to 1 month. Reheat at 200 degrees for 10 minutes.

▶ SERVES 12

tip: Keeping all ingredients—and your mixing bowls!—cold creates a flaky texture in your scones.

featured ingredient

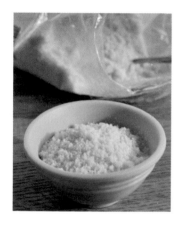

almond flour

To make almond flour, blanched almonds are ground into a fine meal. The flour is great to use in baked goods such as cookies, muffins, or dense cakes. Almond flour lends a sweet flavor and adds protein and healthy fats. It also adds a soft, grainy texture that helps to make cookies crispier and cakes or muffins have a hearty, whole-grain feel. For best results, store almond flour in the freezer.

Pear-Rosemary Bread ⓃⓈ

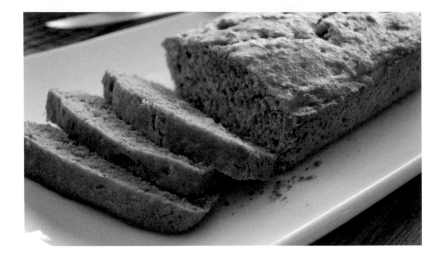

Nonstick (olive oil–flavored) cooking spray

½ cup diced fresh pear

¾ cup spelt flour

½ cup oatmeal flour

1 tablespoon chopped fresh rosemary

½ teaspoon sea salt

2 teaspoons baking powder

2 large eggs

¼ cup agave

¼ cup extra virgin olive oil

⅓ cup chopped walnuts

tip: Refillable spray cans are widely available, so fill with allowable oil and use as nonstick spray.

1. Preheat oven to 350 degrees. Grease an 8 ½" x 4 ½" loaf pan with olive oil spray from a refillable oil mister and set aside.

2. Peel and dice a ripe pear into small pieces and set out on a paper towel to drain excess water.

3. In a large bowl, whisk flours, rosemary, salt, and baking powder, and set aside.

4. In a separate bowl, whisk eggs, agave, and olive oil until well combined. Add the wet ingredients to the flour mixture and stir to combine. Fold in chopped walnuts and drained pears.

5. Spoon batter into prepared loaf pan. Bake 30 to 35 minutes or until cake tester comes out clean.

▶ SERVES 10

featured ingredient

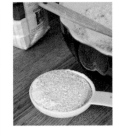

spelt flour

Spelt is an ancient grain related to wheat with a slightly more nutty flavor and a greater amount of nutrients. It can be used as a direct substitution in almost any recipe calling for wheat flour. Although spelt does contain gluten, it does not seem to be a problem for people who cannot tolerate wheat. Spelt can be purchased in a variety of forms, from whole grain to flour, pasta, and bread. Store in the refrigerator to retain the maximum benefits of its nutritional value.

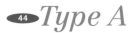

EAT RIGHT FOR YOUR TYPE PERSONALIZED COOKBOOK

Lunch

Each lunch recipe is written to provide a balance between vegetables and varying types of proteins while staying lighter on the complex carbohydrates. Recipes that are more dominantly vegetable or protein have suggestions for a tasty complement of the other.

Adzuki Hummus and Feta Sandwich NS

2 slices brown rice bread

½ teaspoon olive oil

Large-grain sea salt, to taste

2 tablespoons Adzuki Hummus*

1 (¼-inch) slice brick feta cheese

2 thin-sliced artichoke hearts

2 leaves Boston Bibb lettuce

1. Toast bread lightly, just until honey brown, and drizzle one side of each slice with olive oil and a scant sprinkling of sea salt.

2. Spread hummus on the olive oil side of one piece of toast, and top with feta, sliced artichokes, and lettuce leaves. Place the second piece of toast oil side down, and slice in half.

3. Serve immediately.

*See Adzuki Hummus NS recipe (page 153).

▶ SERVES 1

Mushroom and Leek Subs

1. Preheat oven to 375 degrees. Line a baking sheet with parchment paper and set aside.

2. In a large skillet, sauté mushrooms and onions with olive oil for 8 to 10 minutes until mushrooms have released their liquid and onions begin to tenderize. Remove from heat, let cool to room temperature, and drain excess liquid if it exists.

3. Place mushrooms and onions in a food processor with bread crumbs, egg, basil, oregano, and a dash of sea salt. Pulse until ingredients are coarse and combined, not pureed.

4. Use a tablespoon or a small ice cream scoop to form mushroom mixture into balls. Place on prepared baking sheet and bake for 40 minutes or until cooked through.

5. Make sauce: In a large saucepan, heat olive oil over medium-low heat. Sauté onion and garlic for 4 to 5 minutes. Add pimientos and sauté an additional 3 to 4 minutes. Add stock and agave, bring to a boil, and reduce to simmer until mushroom balls are done.

6. Add mushroom balls to sauce and spoon sauce around mushroom to evenly coat.

7. Serve warm topped with mozzarella cheese on toasted buns.

*See Basic Bread Crumbs NS recipe (page 210). See Vegetable Stock NS recipe (page 210).

▶ SERVES 4

3 cups roughly chopped button mushrooms

¼ cup grated onion

2 teaspoons olive oil

1 teaspoon garlic, minced

½ cup bread crumbs*

1 large egg

2 tablespoons basil, chopped

1 tablespoon oregano, chopped

Sea salt, to taste

sauce:

2 teaspoons olive oil

½ cup onions, chopped

1 clove garlic, minced

1 (4.2-oz) jar pimiento, chopped

½ cup Vegetable Stock*

1 teaspoon agave

½ cup basil, chopped

½ cup mozzarella

4 brown rice/millet buns

Fish Fillet Sandwich 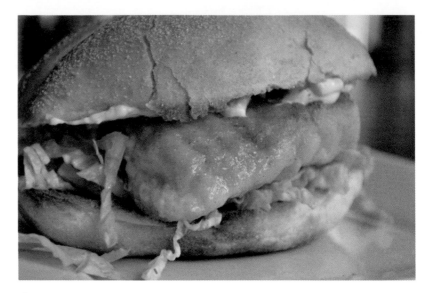 NS

1 pound cod

¼ teaspoon sea salt

1 large egg, slightly beaten

½ cup spelt flour

1 teaspoon garlic powder

1 tablespoon olive oil

4 Ezekiel or spelt buns

1 cup shredded romaine lettuce

sauce:

1 (5.5-oz.) container thick Greek yogurt

1 tablespoon minced onion

Sea salt, to taste

1 tablespoon chopped fresh dill

2 teaspoons lemon zest

1. Season cod with sea salt and slice into 4 individual fillets. In a large, flat-bottomed bowl, add beaten egg, and in a second, add flour and garlic powder. Dip each cod fillet into the egg mixture and then into the flour mixture. Dust off excess flour and place onto a clean plate.

2. In a large, high-sided skillet, heat olive oil over medium heat. Once hot, add fish fillets , keeping 2 inches of space between each. Cook about 4 minutes per side or until center is flaky and opaque.

3. Toast buns and set aside.

4. Combine sauce ingredients in a medium bowl. Spoon yogurt sauce on each half of the bun, and top with romaine and cooked fish.

▶ SERVES 2

tip: Keep an eye on the fish while it cooks to make sure it does not burn. You may need to flip the fish twice to make sure this does not happen. If more oil is needed, add 1 teaspoon at a time.

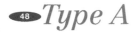

1. Preheat oven or toaster oven to 200 degrees.

2. In a large skillet, heat olive oil over medium heat. Cook bacon for 1 to 2 minutes per side. Drain on paper towels and keep warm in oven; this will help the bacon crisp up further.

3. Add spinach to skillet and cook over medium heat for 1 to 2 minutes with remaining olive oil, just until leaves are wilted.

4. Spread ghee evenly on one side of each piece of bread. Place bacon, spinach, and cheese on unbuttered side of bread and top with a second piece of buttered toast, so that the outer side of each piece is buttered. Toast in a skillet until lightly browned on each side and cheese has melted.

5. Slice in half and serve warm.

▶ SERVES 2

1 teaspoon olive oil

4 strips (nitrate- and preservative-free) turkey bacon

4 cups spinach

4 teaspoons ghee

4 slices oat bread

½ cup shredded mozzarella cheese

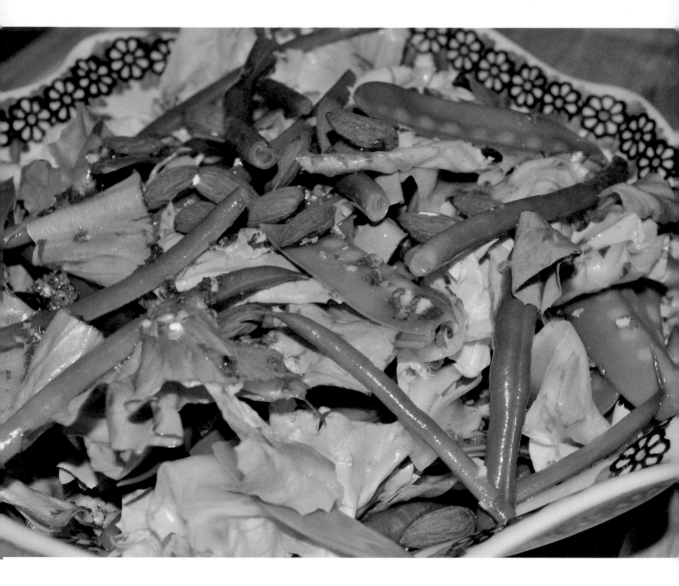

Greens and Beans Salad (NS)

1. Wash escarole and pat dry. Tear escarole in bite-size pieces and place in a large serving bowl. Top with pinto beans, and set aside.

2. Bring a large pot of water to boil. Cook snap peas and string beans for 3 minutes and shock in a large bowl of ice water to stop the cooking process. Lay the peas and beans on a kitchen towel to dry. Add to escarole.

3. In a small bowl, whisk dressing ingredients to combine. Drizzle over salad and serve.

▶ SERVES 4

1 head escarole

½ cup cooked or canned pinto beans, drained and rinsed

2 cups snap peas

4 cups string beans

dressing:

1 tablespoon chopped mint

1 tablespoon fresh lime juice

⅛ teaspoon cumin

1 clove garlic, minced

½ teaspoon honey

¼ cup olive oil

Sea salt, to taste

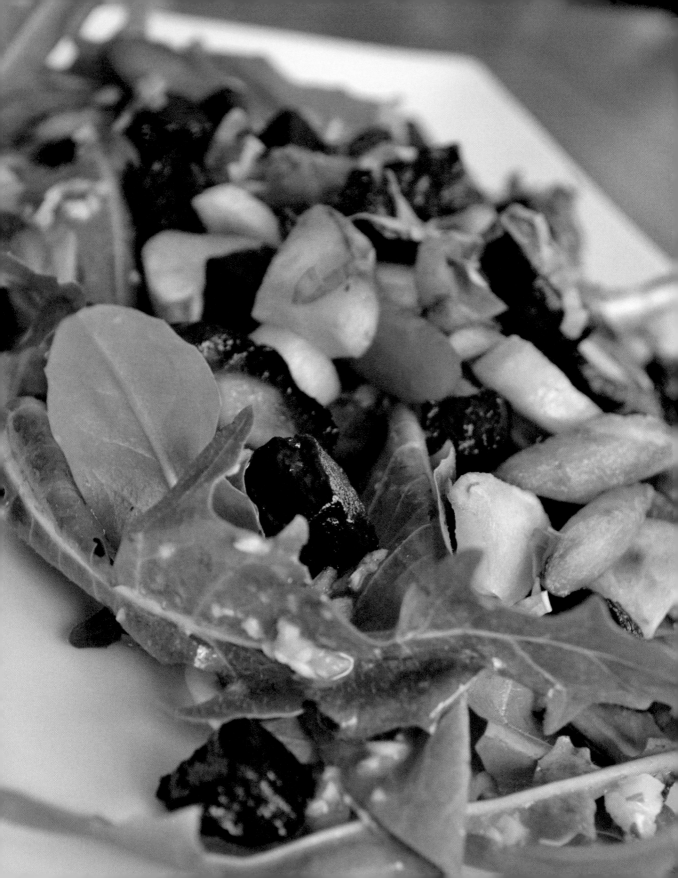

Dandelion Greens with Roasted Roots and Horseradish Dressing (NS)

1. Preheat oven to 375 degrees.

2. Peel beet, carrots, and parsnips. Dice vegetables into ½-inch cubes. Toss with olive oil and season with sea salt. Spread in a single layer on a baking sheet and bake for 55 to 60 minutes, tossing halfway through.

3. To prepare dressing, in a small bowl, whisk horseradish with remaining dressing ingredients.

4. Toss dandelion greens in a large bowl with horseradish dressing, top with roasted vegetables, and serve.

▶ SERVES 4

*If you cannot find tricolored carrots, plain carrots will work just fine.

1 raw beet

3 small, tricolored carrots*

2 medium parsnips

2 teaspoons olive oil

2 bunches dandelion greens

Sea salt, to taste

dressing:

¼ cup fresh, finely grated horseradish

¼ cup olive oil

1 tablespoon fresh basil

2 tablespoons fresh lemon juice

Sea salt, to taste

Roasted-Artichoke Greek Salad (NS)

1 cup artichoke hearts,
quartered

1 teaspoon olive oil

Sea salt, to taste

6 cups torn romaine
lettuce

½ cup crumbled feta
cheese

dressing:

1 tablespoon fresh
oregano

2 tablespoons fresh
squeezed lemon juice

3 tablespoons olive oil

Sea salt, to taste

1. Preheat oven to 375 degrees.

2. Place artichokes on a baking sheet. Drizzle with olive oil, sprinkle with sea salt, and bake for 25 minutes on the top rack of the oven.

3. Remove artichokes from oven and let cool.

4. In a large bowl, whisk dressing ingredients together; set aside.

5. Wash lettuce, and pat dry. Tear into bite-size pieces and place in a serving bowl. Add artichokes, olives, and feta cheese. Drizzle with dressing and toss to combine.

▶ SERVES 4

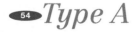

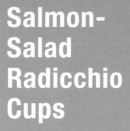

Salmon-Salad Radicchio Cups

1. Start by peeling outer leaves of the radicchio, and discarding the first couple leaves. Continue peeling inner leaves gently, snapping at the base to maintain the integrity of each leaf. Clean with cold water and let dry on a kitchen towel.

2. Flake salmon into a bowl, and add chives, salt, peas, and apples.

3. Make dressing by whisking together honey, oregano, lemon juice and zest, and olive oil. Drizzle over salmon mixture, and spoon salmon into prepared radicchio cups.

▶ SERVES 2

1 head radicchio

½ pound salmon, cooked

3 tablespoons diced chives

½ teaspoon sea salt

½ cup cooked peas

½ cup finely diced apples

1 teaspoon honey

1 tablespoon fresh chopped oregano

Juice and zest of 1 lemon

¼ cup olive oil

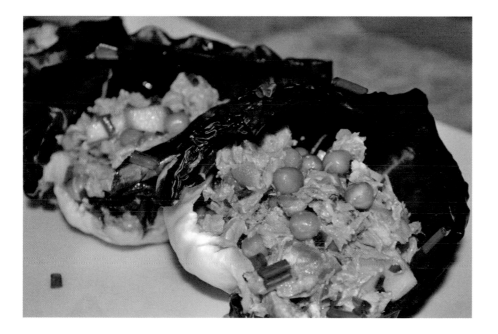

 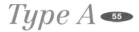

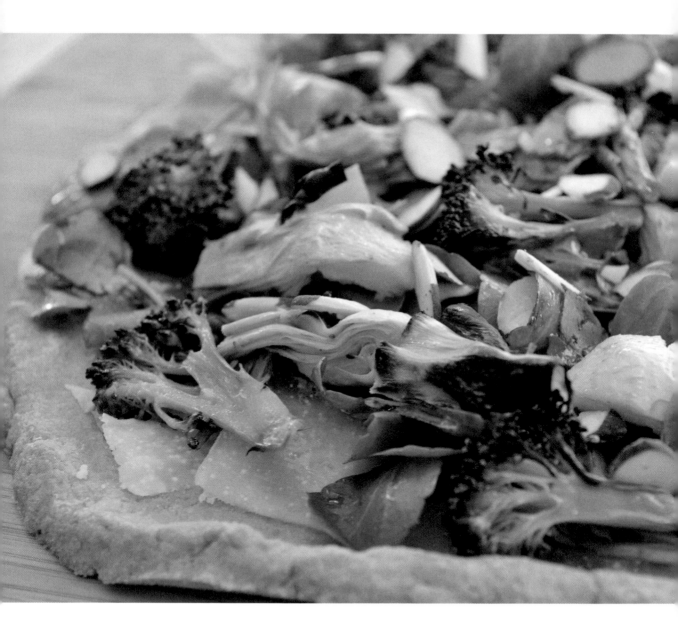

crust:

Store-bought spelt or gluten-free brown rice crust (with allowable grains)

¼ cup shaved, hard goat cheese

2 cups frozen artichoke hearts, thawed

1 head broccoli

1 teaspoon olive oil

Sea salt, to taste

2 cups watercress

¼ cup carrots, shaved

1 tablespoon blanched, slivered almonds

dressing:

1 tablespoon fresh lemon juice

1 teaspoon minced onion

1 tablespoon olive oil

2 teaspoons chopped fresh oregano

1. Preheat oven to 375 degrees.

2. Layer pizza crust with shaved goat cheese and bake for 5 minutes, just until slightly melted. Remove and let cool.

3. Increase oven temperature to 400 degrees. Slice artichokes into quarters, and pat dry. Cut broccoli into bite-size florets, and place on a baking sheet with quartered artichokes. Toss with olive oil and sea salt, and bake for 20 minutes. Broccoli and artichokes will have toasted brown edges and still be brightly colored when done. Let cool.

4. Whisk dressing ingredients together, and toss with watercress, carrots, artichokes, broccoli, and almonds. Top crust with salad mixture and serve cold.

▶ SERVES 4

 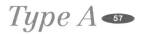

Baked Falafel NS

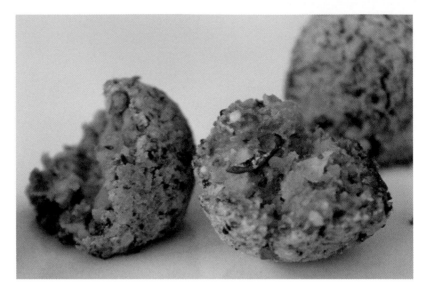

1½ cups dried adzuki beans (not canned or precooked)

1 tablespoon olive oil, divided

½ cup chopped parsley

2 tablespoons oat flour

1 cup chopped onion

2 cloves garlic, minced

¼ teaspoon coriander

¼ teaspoon cumin

½ teaspoon sea salt

1. Soak dry beans overnight in cold water. Drain and rinse.

2. Boil presoaked beans for 30 minutes. Drain and rinse. Beans will not be completely cooked. Leaving them slightly firm will help falafel's texture. Set beans in a single layer on a paper towel to dry.

3. Preheat oven to 350 degrees. Brush baking sheet with ½ tablespoon oil, and set aside.

4. In a food processor, add beans and parsley, flour, onion, garlic, coriander, cumin, and salt. Pulse until ingredients form a thick paste. Use a tablespoon to scoop mixture into the palm of your hand, roll into balls, and place on prepared baking sheet. Continue until all of the mixture has been used. Brush remaining olive oil on the tops of falafel balls and bake in the oven for 25 minutes.

5. Increase oven temperature to 400 degrees and bake an additional 15 minutes.

6. Serve on top of Roasted-Artichoke Greek Salad (page 54).

▶ SERVES 4

EAT RIGHT FOR YOUR TYPE PERSONALIZED COOKBOOK

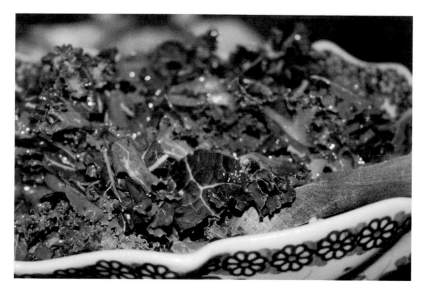

Raw Kale Salad with Zesty Lime Dressing NS

1 bunch kale

2 teaspoons olive oil

1 large white onion, sliced

½ cup raisins

dressing:

2 tablespoons olive oil

2 limes, juiced

1 clove garlic, minced

⅛ teaspoon ground cumin

Sea salt, to taste

1. Wash kale and dry on kitchen towels. Strip kale off the woody stems by holding the stem with one hand and wrapping finger and thumb of the other hand around the stem and pulling quickly down. Discard stems and tear leaves into bite-size pieces. Place in a large bowl and set aside.

2. In a skillet, heat olive oil over medium heat. Add onion, and sauté for 3 to 4 minutes. Add raisins and continue cooking for 5 minutes. Remove from heat and toss with raw kale.

3. In a small bowl, whisk dressing ingredients. Drizzle over kale salad and toss to coat.

4. Serve with leftover or chilled, baked salmon, roasted chicken, or beans for added protein.

▶ SERVES 6

 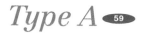

Crunchy Kohlrabi Spring Rolls with Sweet Cherry Dip (NS)

spring rolls:

1 kohlrabi, bulb and leaves

3 small tricolored carrots

2 teaspoons olive oil

¼ cup finely chopped onion

¼ cup julienned fresh basil

Sea salt, to taste

4 large rice paper wraps

sweet cherry dip:

⅓ cup (no sugar added) cherry jam

1 tablespoon fresh grated ginger

1 tablespoon finely diced onion

1 teaspoon agave

Juice of half a lemon

Sea salt, to taste

1. Prepare kohlrabi by pulling leaves off stalks, then wash and let dry on a kitchen towel. Peel bulb and slice off tough top and bottom. Slice into thin matchsticks and set aside. Peel and slice carrots in the same fashion.

2. In a skillet, heat olive oil over medium heat. Sauté onion for 5 to 6 minutes. Add kohlrabi greens and sauté an additional 2 minutes. Remove from heat and let cool.

3. Add carrots, kohlrabi, and basil to sautéed vegetables; toss to combine.

4. Pour hot water halfway up a large, flat-bottomed bowl. One at a time, submerge rice paper wraps in water until they soften and become malleable. This will take about 30 seconds. Rice paper will be delicate so be gentle! Place rice wrap on a plate or cutting board, and spoon about 2 tablespoons of the vegetable mixture down the center of the rice paper. Roll the sides over the vegetables first, pull the top over the vegetables and continue to roll over itself. Slice in half. Repeat until all of the filling is gone.

5. In a small saucepan, combine all sauce ingredients. Stir 1 to 2 minutes until warmed through and melted together.

6. Serve wraps with cherry dip.

▶ SERVES 2

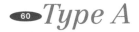

EAT RIGHT FOR YOUR TYPE PERSONALIZED COOKBOOK

featured ingredient

kohlrabi

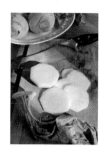

It looks like a root, but actually grows above ground and is abundant with nutritional value for Type As. The bulb sprouts long stems with leafy tops, which are also edible. Kohlrabi can be eaten raw or cooked.

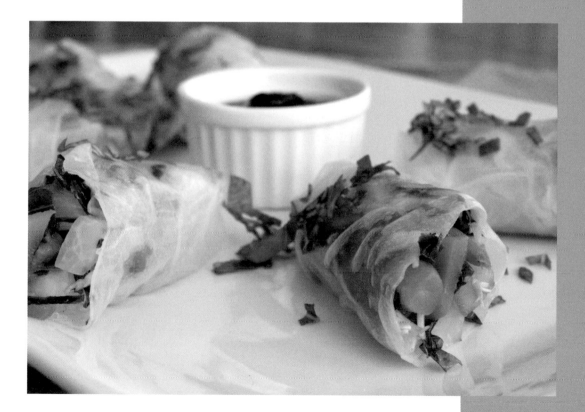

Feta, Spinach, and Broccolini Pie NS

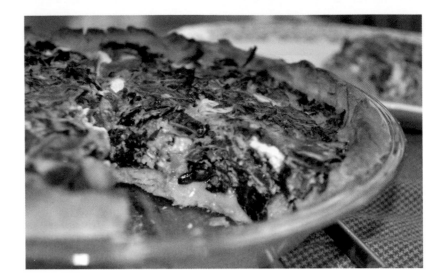

crust:

1 cup spelt flour plus more for rolling

¼ teaspoon sea salt

4 tablespoons chilled ghee

4–5 tablespoons ice cold water

filling:

2 teaspoons olive oil

4 cups baby spinach

½ cup diced white onion

2 cups chopped broccolini

1 cup crumbled feta cheese

2 large eggs

⅓ cup Vegetable Stock*

2 tablespoons fresh thyme

Sea salt, to taste

1. Preheat oven to 375 degrees.

2. Combine flour and salt in a large bowl. Cut cold ghee into small pieces, and add to flour mixture. Using a crossing motion with two butter knives or a pastry cutter, incorporate ghee into the flour until the mixture resembles coarse corn meal. Add water, 1 tablespoon at a time, until the dough comes together but is not sticky. Gather dough in your hands, and knead until dough becomes smooth and pliable, being careful not to overwork the dough. Small pieces of ghee should still be visible. Cover with plastic wrap and refrigerate dough for 1 hour.

3. Roll dough out on a floured surface until about 12 inches in diameter and approximately 1/8-inch thick. Gently press the dough into a 9-inch pie plate, and pinch edges between two fingers to create pleated edges.

4. Par-bake crust for 15 minutes. ("Par-bake" means that you are partially baking the crust before adding the filling.)

5. While the crust bakes, make filling. In a large skillet over medium heat, heat olive oil. Sauté spinach, onion, and broccolini for 4 minutes or just until vegetables are tender. Remove vegetables and place into a large bowl, toss with feta, and let cool.

6. In a separate bowl, whisk eggs, stock, thyme, and salt. Pour over cooled vegetables and mix to combine.

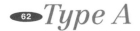

7. Pour filling into par-baked spelt pie crust and bake 30 minutes or until filling is firm.

8. Serve warm or cold (if serving cold, let cool and then place in refrigerator until ready to eat).

*See Vegetable Stock NS recipe (page 210).

▶ SERVES 6

featured ingredient

broccolini

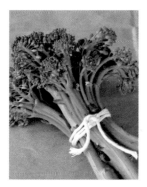

Broccolini looks like an elongated and tender version of its look-alike, broccoli. Broccolini has a slightly more mild taste and is much more palatable when sautéed, roasted, or grilled. If cooked simply, it pairs best with olive oil and garlic. It is often confused with rappini or broccoli rabe, which has a much more bitter taste and is less appealing to most people.

Fava Bean Stew (NS)

2 teaspoons olive oil

1 cup diced onion

1 celery root, peeled and cut into ¼-inch dice

2 cups ½-inch diced sweet potato

4 cups fava beans, rinsed and drained

1½ cups Vegetable Stock*

1 clove garlic

1 sprig sage

4 sprigs thyme

1 teaspoon sea salt

2 cups snow peas

1. In a Dutch oven, heat olive oil over medium heat. Add onions and celery root and sauté for 4 to 5 minutes. Add sweet potato, and sauté an additional 2 to 3 minutes. Add beans, stock, garlic, sage, thyme, and salt, and bring to a gentle boil.

2. Reduce heat, cover, and simmer 30 minutes.

3. Add snow peas and cook an additional 5 minutes.

4. Serve warm.

*See Vegetable Stock NS recipe (page 210).

▶ SERVES 4

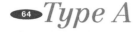

Dinner

The bulk of the recipes in this book are in this section. Here you will find a variety of dishes from pastas to seafood, all-in-one dishes, and so on. Most of the recipes are simple to make, but others take a bit more time to prepare. Hopefully these dishes inspire you to take some time to enjoy delicious, wholesome food for yourself and your family.

Mac and Cheese with Roasted Vegetables NS

1 bunch leeks

1 large head broccoli

5 sprigs thyme

1 tablespoon olive oil

Sea salt, to taste

1 tablespoon plus 2 teaspoons ghee, divided

⅔ cup bread crumbs*

2 tablespoons spelt flour

2 cups Vegetable Stock*

1 cup almond milk

2 sprigs fresh sage

1 pound spelt or brown rice pasta

1 cup shredded mozzarella cheese

½ cup cubed fresh mozzarella cheese

1. Preheat oven to 375 degrees.

2. Slice leeks down the middle and rinse thoroughly under water to remove all of the dirt between the layers. Let dry on a kitchen towel. Cut leeks into 1-inch half-moon shapes. Cut broccoli into bite-size pieces.

Strip thyme sprigs of leaves. Line vegetables on a baking sheet, drizzle with olive oil and thyme, and sprinkle with salt. Bake for 30 minutes, until vegetables are tender and slightly browned around the edges. Set aside.

3. Melt 2 teaspoons of ghee, toss with bread crumbs and a pinch of sea salt, and set aside.

4. Make a roux by melting remaining 1 tablespoon of ghee in a saucepan and whisking in flour until well combined into a paste. Gradually add stock and milk to flour mixture, each time whisking after each addition until smooth and without lumps. Add sage and bring to a boil, whisking constantly. Reduce to a simmer, and cook until the roux thickens, about 10 minutes. Add salt, to taste.

5. Cook pasta according to package instructions. If using brown rice pasta, only cook 8 minutes (slightly less than half of package instructions), drain, and pour into casserole dish. Toss with roasted vegetables. Cover pasta with sauce and shredded cheese and mix to incorporate. Top with reserved bread crumbs and ½ cup cubed fresh mozzarella.

6. Bake 20 to 25 minutes, until hot and bubbling and the bread crumbs are golden brown and toasted.

*See Basic Bread Crumbs NS recipe (page 210). See Vegetable Stock NS recipe (page 210).

▶ SERVES 6

Spring Pesto Pasta NS

1. Preheat oven to 375 degrees.

2. Snap asparagus spears close to the bottom and discard the woody stems. Cut into bite-size pieces and place in a large bowl. Tear 1½ bunches of kale into large, bite-size pieces. Place in bowl with asparagus and toss with 2 teaspoons olive oil and a pinch of salt.

3. Place vegetables on a baking sheet and bake for 12 minutes or until tender and edges of kale are slightly crispy.

4. Cook pasta according to package instructions. If using brown rice pasta, cook 4 to 5 minutes short of package instructions.

5. Tear remaining kale into bite-size pieces; you'll have about 2 ½ cups. Combine with ½ cup olive oil, lemon juice, walnuts, garlic, salt, and pepper in a food processor, and pulse until smooth. Spoon into a bowl and set aside.

6. Cook bacon in a skillet with remaining 1 teaspoon olive oil until crispy, about 2 minutes per side. Wrap in a paper towel and keep warm in the oven on 200 until ready to serve, to make bacon extra crispy.

7. Drain pasta, and place in a large pasta bowl. Toss immediately with pesto, peas, and roasted vegetables.

8. Sprinkle with crumbled bacon and serve warm.

▶ SERVES 6

1 bunch asparagus

2 large bunches kale, divided

½ cup plus 3 teaspoons olive oil

Sea salt, to taste

1 pound spelt or brown rice pasta

1 lemon, juice and zest, divided

½ cup walnuts

2 cloves garlic, minced

3 slices turkey bacon

2 cups cooked peas

Pumpkin Gnocchi with Basil-Cranberry Sauce NS

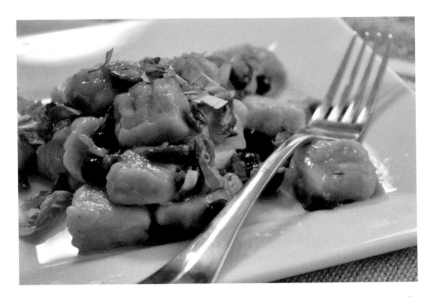

2 cups organic canned pumpkin

¾ cup brown rice flour

¼ cup millet flour

1 teaspoon sea salt

1 large egg, beaten

¼ teaspoon fresh ground nutmeg

sauce:

1 tablespoon olive oil

1 teaspoon ghee

¼ cup finely diced shallots

½ cup Vegetable Stock*

1 tablespoon lemon juice

¼ cup dried cranberries

½ cup torn fresh basil

1. In a large bowl, combine gnocchi ingredients. Use your hands to form lightly into a dough ball. If the dough is too sticky, sprinkle more brown rice flour over the dough. Grab a handful of dough at a time and roll on a floured surface into long, ¾-inch-thick cylinders. Repeat with remaining dough.

2. Use a sharp knife to slice the cylinders into 1-inch pieces. Roll each piece gently over the back of a fork, to make indentations in the gnocchi.

3. Bring a large pot of salted water to a gentle boil. Drop gnocchi into the water in batches; do not crowd the pot. The gnocchi will float to the top when they are finished cooking, about 2 to 3 minutes. Remove to a baking sheet until all gnocchi has been cooked.

4. Heat olive oil and ghee in a large skillet over medium heat. Sauté shallots for 2 to 3 minutes, then add stock, lemon juice, and cranberries.

5. Toss gnocchi with sauce just to coat. Garnish with basil and serve warm.

*See Vegetable Stock recipe NS (page 210).

▶ SERVES 4

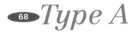

EAT RIGHT FOR YOUR TYPE PERSONALIZED COOKBOOK

Pasta Carbonara with Crispy Kale (NS)

1 pound spelt or brown rice pasta

2 teaspoons olive oil

½ cup onions, diced

4 slices turkey bacon

3 cups sliced Swiss chard

3 cups sliced red kale

2 large eggs

2 large egg yolks

¼ cup soy or almond milk

½ cup ricotta cheese

Sea salt, to taste

1. Cook pasta according to package instructions. If using brown rice pasta, cook 4 minutes short of package cooking time. Drain, reserve ½ cup pasta water, and set aside.

2. Heat olive oil in a large, high-sided skillet over medium heat. Sauté onions for 4 to 5 minutes. Add turkey bacon and sauté until browned. Remove turkey bacon, and set aside. In the same pan, add Swiss chard and kale, and sauté until tender, about 3 to 4 minutes. Crumble bacon, return to skillet, and reduce heat to low.

3. In a bowl, whisk together eggs, yolks, milk, ricotta cheese, and salt. Slowly pour reserved pasta cooking water into the egg mixture to temper the eggs. Remove the skillet from the heat, and toss in freshly cooked pasta as you pour over egg mixture. The heat from the pasta will gently cook the eggs and create a sauce.

4. Serve immediately.

▶ SERVES 6

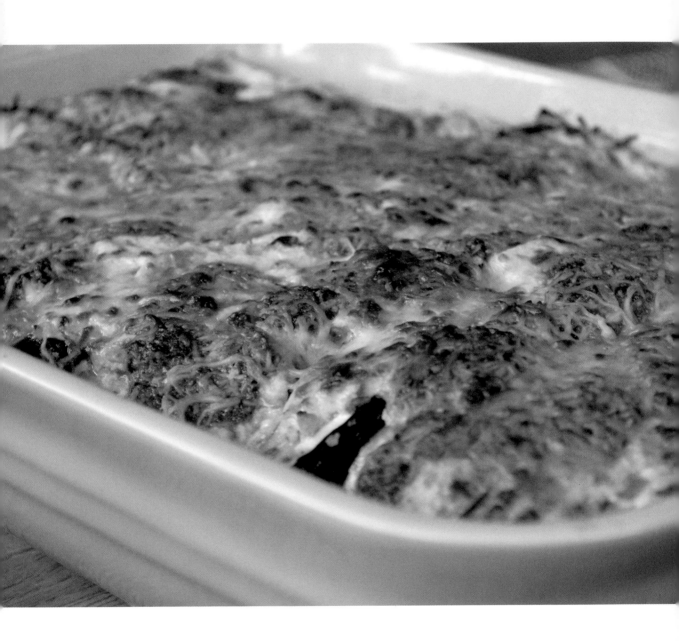

Veggie Lasagna NS

1. Preheat oven to 375 degrees.

2. Trim ends off zucchini and slice into 4 long pieces, resembling thick lasagna noodles, about ¼-inch thick.

3. Line zucchini and portabella mushrooms in a single layer on baking sheets. Drizzle evenly with 2 tablespoons olive oil and 1 teaspoon sea salt. Roast on the top shelf of the oven for 20 minutes.

4. Heat remaining 2 teaspoons olive oil in a medium skillet over medium heat. Sauté onion for 8 to 10 minutes, until tender and translucent. Add spinach and sauté 1 minute, just until spinach wilts. Remove from heat.

5. In a large bowl, stir together ricotta cheese, walnuts, egg, cloves and reserved spinach mixture. Set aside.

6. Remove vegetables from the oven and let cool. Reduce oven temperature to 350 degrees.

7. Place all pesto ingredients in a blender and puree until smooth.

8. Assemble lasagna by layering a thin layer of pesto in the bottom of a 9" x 11" baking dish. Top with a layer of roasted zucchini, a layer of ricotta mixture, ½ cup mozzarella cheese, pesto, mushrooms, ricotta, pesto, remaining zucchini, remaining ricotta, remaining pesto, and remaining mozzarella cheese.

9. Bake for 25 minutes until the cheese is melted, and slightly browned on the top.

10. Serve warm.

▶ SERVES 6

5 medium zucchini

6 portabella mushrooms

2 tablespoons plus 2 teaspoons olive oil, divided

1½ teaspoons sea salt, divided

1 cup finely diced onion

4 cups packed baby spinach

2 cups part-skim ricotta cheese

½ cup finely chopped walnuts

1 large egg

Dash ground cloves

1 cup shredded mozzarella cheese

pesto:

2 cups packed baby spinach

2 cups packed basil

½ teaspoon sea salt

2 cloves garlic

¼ cup lemon juice

¼ cup olive oil

¼ cup walnuts

2 tablespoons water

Grilled Radicchio and Walnut-Spinach Pesto 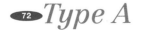 NS

infused oil:

½ lemon, zest only

⅓ cup olive oil

⅛ teaspoon mustard powder

½ teaspoon cumin seeds

2 cloves garlic, smashed

pesto:

¼ cup plus 2 tablespoons toasted almonds, divided

2 tablespoons olive oil

2 tablespoons chopped fresh sage

1 cup chopped spinach

2 tablespoons lemon juice

1 teaspoon lemon zest

½ teaspoon sea salt

1 tablespoon water

¾ pound spinach spelt pasta

2 heads radicchio

1. In a small skillet, combine all infused oil ingredients. Cook over low heat for 15 minutes. Remove from heat and set aside.*

2. In a food processor or mini-chopper, combine pesto ingredients: ¼ cup almonds, olive oil, sage, spinach, lemon juice, lemon zest, sea salt, and water. Pulse until mixture is pureed and resembles a thick sauce.

3. Bring a large pot of water to boil. Cook pasta according to package instructions.

4. While the pasta cooks, heat grill pan over medium and brush with infused oil. Peel outer layers of radicchio and cut them in quarters. Brush each quarter with infused olive oil and grill about 1 minute per side, or until radicchio begins to become tender and slightly wilted.

5. Drain pasta and toss with pesto in a large serving bowl. Top with grilled radicchio and remaining toasted almonds. Serve immediately.

▶ SERVES 4

tip: Store infused oil in a sealed, glass container in a cool, dry place for up to 1 week. Great on salads or drizzled over toast.

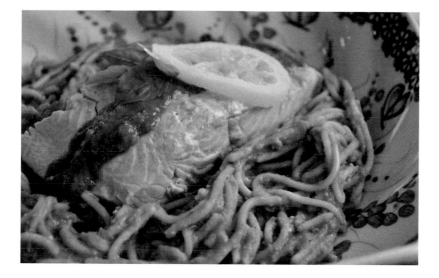

Noodles with Poached Salmon and Basil Cream NS

2 cups Vegetable Stock*
2 cups water
1 lemon, sliced
1½ pounds salmon
1 pound spelt pasta
Spicy mustard, for serving, optional

basil cream:
2 cups spinach
1 cup basil
1 clove garlic, minced
1 cup northern beans, rinsed and drained
2 teaspoons lemon zest
½ cup Vegetable Stock*

1. Fill a high-sided skillet with stock, water, and lemon slices. Bring to a simmer and add salmon. Cover and cook 12 to 15 minutes.

2. In the meantime, bring a large pot of water to boil and cook pasta according to package instructions.

3. Puree all sauce ingredients in a food processor or blender.

4. Drain pasta and toss with all but ¼ cup of the basil sauce. Top with salmon and drizzle with remaining sauce and spicy mustard, if desired.

5. Serve immediately.

*See Vegetable Stock recipe NS (page 210).

▶ SERVES 4

Salmon–Black Bean Cakes with Cilantro–Cream Sauce NS

1 pound wild-caught salmon, cooked

1 cup cooked black beans, rinsed and drained

1 teaspoon chopped scallions

1 teaspoon fresh rosemary

1 teaspoon fresh thyme

Sea salt, to taste

1 large egg, slightly beaten

½ cup bread crumbs*

2 teaspoons olive oil

sauce:

2 tablespoons walnuts

2 tablespoons olive oil

2 tablespoons hot water

¼ cup fresh cilantro

Sea salt, to taste

1. Flake cooked salmon into a bowl, and carefully remove any bones. Add beans, scallions, rosemary, thyme, and sea salt. Gently stir in egg and bread crumbs.

2. Form salmon mixture into patties the size of a baseball. Repeat until all of the salmon mixture is used.

3. Heat olive oil in a large skillet over medium heat. Cook salmon patties for 3 to 4 minutes. Turn and cook an additional 3 to 4 minutes.

4. In a food processor, chop walnuts until they form a paste. With the processor running, add olive oil and water until mixture becomes creamy. Add cilantro and salt and blend until smooth.

5. Serve salmon cakes warm, drizzled with cilantro-cream sauce.

*See Basic Bread Crumbs recipe NS (page 210).

▶ SERVES 4

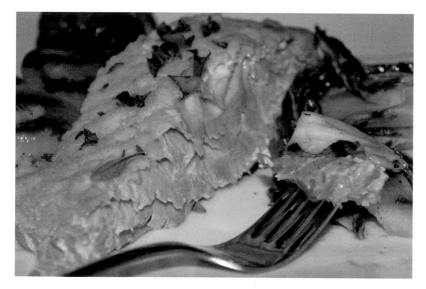

Lemon-Ginger Salmon NS

1 pound wild-salmon fillets

2 teaspoons olive oil, divided

½ teaspoon sea salt

Zest of 1 lemon

1 tablespoon lemon juice

2 tablespoons fresh grated ginger

1 teaspoon honey

1. Preheat oven to 400 degrees.

2. Rub salmon filletls with 1 teaspoon olive oil and season with sea salt.

3. In a small bowl, mix the zest of 1 lemon, lemon juice, remaining 1 teaspoon olive oil, ginger, and honey until combined. Brush evenly over the top of salmon.

4. Bake for 10 to 12 minutes.

5. Serve with Grilled Sesame-Ginger Bok Choy NS (page 121).

▶ SERVES 2

 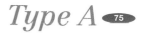

Baked Mahimahi with Crunchy Fennel Salad NS

1 pound mahimahi
steaks

⅛ teaspoon ground
coriander

1 teaspoon fresh lemon
zest

¼ teaspoon sea salt

fennel salad:

2 teaspoons chopped
parsley

2 teaspoons olive oil

Sea salt, to taste

1 teaspoon lemon zest

2 teaspoons lemon juice

2 cups thinly sliced
fennel

1 cup thinly sliced
Granny Smith apples

1. Preheat oven to 350 degrees.

2. Season mahimahi with coriander, lemon zest, and sea salt. Bake for 12 to 15 minutes or until fish is flaky and white.

3. While the seafood bakes, whisk parsley, olive oil, sea salt, to taste, lemon zest, and juice in the bottom of a bowl. Add fennel and apple, and toss with dressing.

4. Plate fish and top with fennel salad. Serve immediately.

▶ SERVES 2

tip: Don't rush when you have a sharp knife in your hand, no matter what the circumstance, and remember to tuck your fingers so your knuckles stick out slightly beyond the curl of your fingertips, so that the knife can glide harmlessly across your food, using your knuckles as a safety guide.

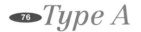

Seared Tuna with Fig and Basil Chutney NS

1. Drizzle each tuna steak with 1 teaspoon olive oil and sprinkle both sides with sea salt. Set aside.

2. In a small saucepan, whisk fig jam, basil, lemon zest, juice, and remaining 1 teaspoon olive oil. Warm over low heat while tuna cooks.

3. Heat a skillet over medium and when it is hot, spray with non-stick olive oil cooking spray. Sear tuna for 1½ minutes per side. If you do not like your tuna rare inside, cook 2 to 3 minutes per side or until desired doneness.

4. Top with fig and basil chutney and serve.

▶ SERVES 2

1 pound wild-caught tuna steaks

2 tablespoons plus 1 teaspoon olive oil

½ teaspoon sea salt

¼ cup fig jam

2 tablespoons chopped fresh basil

2 teaspoons lemon zest

2 tablespoons lemon juice

 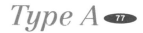

Parchment-Baked Snapper (NS)

1 pound snapper (4 fillets)

½ teaspoon sea salt

2 teaspoons chopped fresh oregano

2 cloves garlic, minced

½ cup diced green olives (NS omit olives)

1 cup thinly sliced fennel

1 cup thinly sliced red onion

1 tablespoon olive oil

1. Preheat oven to 350 degrees.

2. Cut 4 pieces of parchment paper into about 12-inch–15-inch sections. Fold parchment pieces in half and cut into a large heart shape, like cutting out a valentine. Place snapper in one half of the parchment heart, and season with salt, oregano, and garlic.

3. Top with olives, sliced fennel, and red onion, and drizzle each fillet with 1 teaspoon olive oil.

4. Wrap fish in parchment paper by folding edges over: start at the top of the heart to roll and crease the edges. Crimp ends of parchment paper to seal the sides and bake on a baking sheet for 12 to 15 minutes or until snapper flakes easily with a fork.

▶ SERVES 4

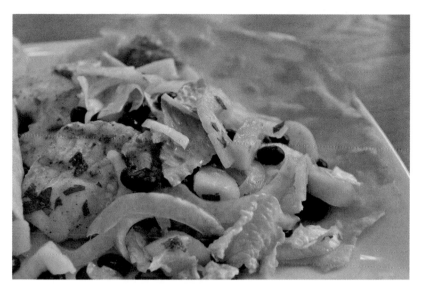

Fish Tacos with Bean and Crunchy Fennel Slaw

1 pound cod

½ teaspoon garlic powder

⅛ teaspoon cumin

½ teaspoon salt

¼ teaspoon paprika

2 teaspoons olive oil

8 soft corn-only taco shells (NS substitute small spelt wrap)

fennel slaw:

1 fennel bulb, finely sliced

1 tablespoon chopped fresh mint

½ teaspoon lime zest

1 lime, sections and remaining juice

2 teaspoons olive oil

½ cup pineapple, small dice

¼ teaspoon salt

1. Slice fish into bite-size pieces and place in a small bowl with garlic powder, cumin, salt, paprika, and olive oil. Toss gently. Marinate in the refrigerator at least 20 minutes.

2. Place all fennel slaw ingredients in a large bowl and toss to combine. Set aside in refrigerator until ready to eat. (Letting the slaw sit while fish is cooking enables the flavors to combine and textures to soften slightly.)

3. Remove fish from the refrigerator. Heat a grill pan over medium-high heat and brush with olive oil. Grill fish 2 to 3 minutes per side.

4. Warm taco shells by dry toasting them in a large skillet for 1 minute per side over medium heat. (NS, warm small spelt wraps by wrapping with damp paper towels and keeping in the toaster oven on 150 degrees for 5 minutes. Be VERY careful not to let the paper towel get close to the burners and keep an eye on it so the paper towels don't dry out.) When removed from the pan, immediately wrap tacos in a kitchen cloth to keep warm.

5. To assemble tacos, place taco on a plate and top with fish and fennel slaw.

6. Serve warm.

▶ SERVES 4

Type A 79

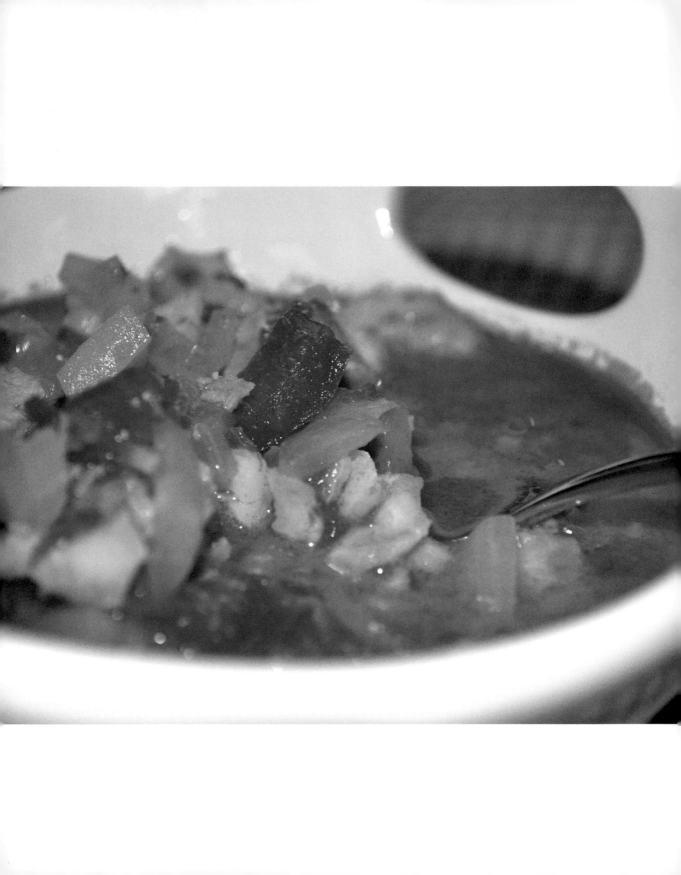

1. Soak wakame in a bowl of cold water for 10 minutes.

2. In a stockpot, sauté leeks and fennel in olive oil for 4 to 5 minutes over medium heat. Season with turmeric, fennel seeds, bay leaves, and salt, to taste.

3. Drain wakame, rinse, and immediately add to stockpot.

4. Drain cans of pimiento and pat dry. Puree in a food processor until very smooth. Add puree and 2 bay leaves to sautéed vegetables in the stockpot with stock and water. Let simmer 30 minutes.

5. While the stew simmers, dice cod and salmon into bite-size pieces. After the stew simmers for 30 minutes, add the seafood and okra and let cook an additional 10 minutes or until seafood is cooked through.

6. Serve warm.

*See Vegetable Stock NS recipe (page 210).

¼ cup wakame

2 teaspoons olive oil

1 cup diced leeks

1 bulb diced fennel

½ teaspoon turmeric

½ teaspoon fennel seeds

2 bay leaves

Sea salt, to taste

2 (6½-oz.) cans pimiento

1 cup Vegetable Stock*

¾ pound cod

½ pound wild-caught salmon

2 cups diced okra

▶ SERVES 4

featured ingredient

wakame

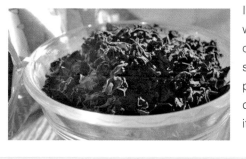

If you've had miso soup, you've most likely eaten wakame. Wakame is a nutrient-rich seaweed cultivated off the coast of Japan, and adds a briny finish to soups, stews, and even salads. It is most often dehydrated (as pictured) for distribution, but once soaked, it returns to its dark-green color and velvety texture. With its mild flavor, it is a perfect way to begin adding seaweed to your diet!

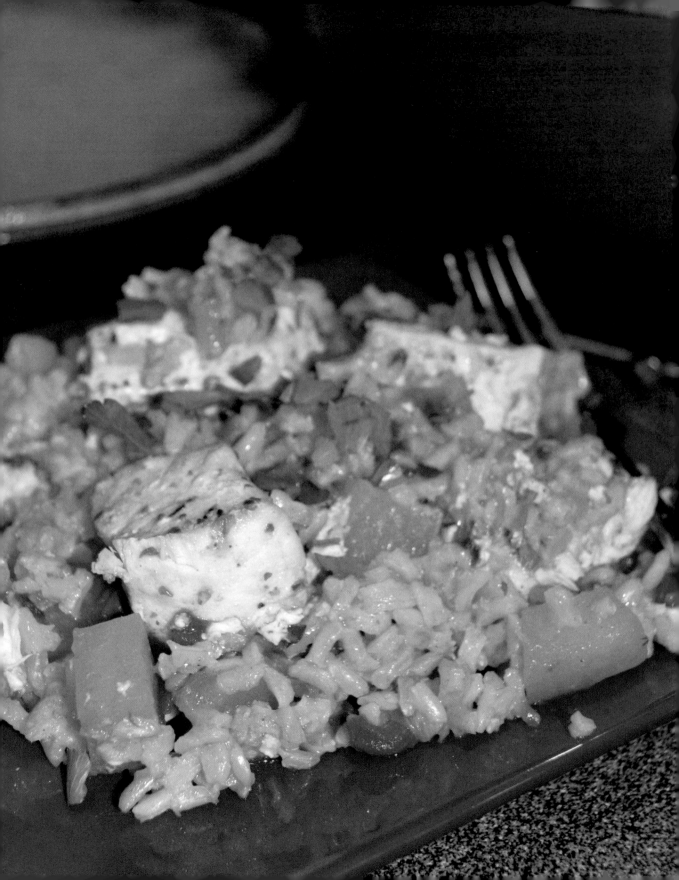

1. Preheat oven to 350 degrees.

2. Heat 2 teaspoons olive oil in a large Dutch oven or paella pan set over medium heat. Sauté onions and rutabaga for 6 to 7 minutes. Add pimientos, parsley, and garlic, and sauté for an additional 4 to 5 minutes. Remove from pan, and set aside.

3. Add remaining 1 teaspoon olive oil to the same pan and toast rice for 2 minutes, stirring constantly. Add saffron, sea salt, and paprika.

4. Return all vegetables to the Dutch oven, and stir to combine with rice. Add stock, water, bay leaf, and fresh oregano. Bring to a simmer, and cover. Place in preheated oven and cook for 45 minutes.

5. While the paella cooks, dice snapper and cod into 1-inch pieces, and toss fish with dried oregano and sea salt to taste.

6. Remove paella from oven, and add seafood pieces. Bake an additional 12 minutes.

7. Seafood should be flaky and opaque when fully cooked. Rice will be fluffy and tender.

8. Serve warm.

*See Vegetable Stock NS recipe (page 210).

▶ SERVES 6

3 teaspoons olive oil, divided

2 cups diced yellow onion

1 cup diced rutabaga

2 (6½-oz.) cans whole pimiento

¼ cup chopped parsley

2 teaspoons garlic, minced

1½ cups long-grain brown rice

15 threads saffron

Sea salt, to taste

1 teaspoon paprika

2 cups Vegetable Stock*

1 cup water

1 bay leaf

2 teaspoons fresh oregano

¾ pound red snapper fillet

¾ pound cod fillet

1 teaspoon dried oregano

Green Tea–Poached Chicken (NS)

4 cups water, plus 1 tablespoon water

8 green tea bags

1 pound chicken breasts, cut into 4 pieces

½ lemon, sliced

½ teaspoon sea salt

1 cup fresh parsley

Juice from ½ lemon

3 tablespoons olive oil

1 clove garlic

1 tablespoon water

1. In a high-sided skillet, bring 4 cups water to a boil and steep the tea bags for 3 minutes. Reduce heat to medium and add chicken breasts, lemon slices, and sea salt. Cover and let cook 18 to 20 minutes, or until the internal temperature reaches 165 degrees.

2. Puree parsley, lemon juice, olive oil, garlic, and remaining 1 tablespoon water in a food processor until very smooth.

3. Serve chicken warm, topped with parsley oil.

▶ SERVES 4

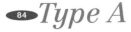

1. Season chicken thighs with salt and place in a sealable glass container. Add olive oil and garlic. Cover, and refrigerate at least 1 hour to marinate. Remove from fridge and let come to room temperature before using.

2. Blend all pesto ingredients in a food processor until smooth and combined. Set aside.

3. Heat a grill pan over medium and brush with olive oil. Slice chicken into medallions and grill 5 to 6 minutes on each side.

4. Top with pesto, and serve with Forbidden Black Rice Risotto.*

*See Forbidden Black Rice Risotto NS recipe (page 143).

▶ SERVES 4

1 pound skinless, organic chicken thighs
Sea salt, to taste
½ cup olive oil
3 cloves garlic, chopped

pesto:
½ cup fresh spinach
1 bunch fresh mint
1 teaspoon minced garlic
¼ cup extra virgin olive oil
½ teaspoon sea salt
Juice of 1 lemon
¼ cup raw walnuts

 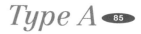

Chicken Pot Pie with Crunchy Topping NS

filling:

2 teaspoons olive oil

1 cup pearl onions

1 cup diced baby carrots

1 cup sweet peas

1 cup chopped okra

2 tablespoons oat flour

3¼ cups chicken broth

1½ pounds roasted chicken breast

½ teaspoon saffron threads

½ teaspoon dry mustard

topping:

2 cups diced Jerusalem artichoke

1 teaspoon olive oil

½ cup bread crumbs*

2 tablespoons sesame seeds

2 teaspoons ghee, melted

crust:

Spelt or whole wheat store-bought crust (containing allowable grains)

1. Preheat oven to 375 degrees.

2. Heat 2 teaspoons olive oil in a Dutch oven over medium heat. Sauté onions, carrots, peas, and okra for 5 minutes. Sprinkle flour over vegetables and add broth, stirring to prevent lumps. Add roasted chicken, saffron, and dry mustard, stirring to combine. Cover and let cook 15 minutes, stirring occasionally.

3. In a large skillet, heat 1 teaspoon olive oil over medium heat. Sauté Jerusalem artichokes for 3 to 4 minutes. Remove and toss with bread crumbs and sesame seeds. Drizzle with melted ghee.

4. Spoon chicken filling into spelt crust, and top with artichoke mixture. Place in the oven, and bake 25 to 30 minutes, until crust is brown and top is bubbling.

5. Serve warm.

*See Basic Bread crumbs NS recipe (page 210).

▶ SERVES 8

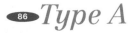

featured ingredient

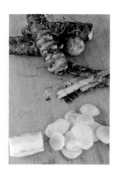

jerusalem artichoke

Crisp and crunchy, Jerusalem artichoke is a root vegetable with a beautiful yellow flower resembling a sunflower. They have a slightly sweet, nutty flavor and can be used similar to potatoes or sliced thinly and fried. Neutral to most Type As, Jerusalem artichokes are a fun, tasty new vegetable to get your hands on.

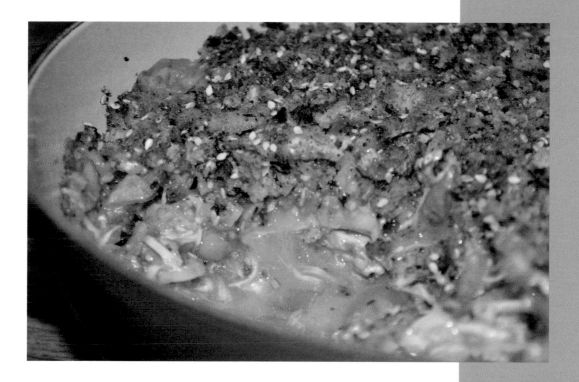

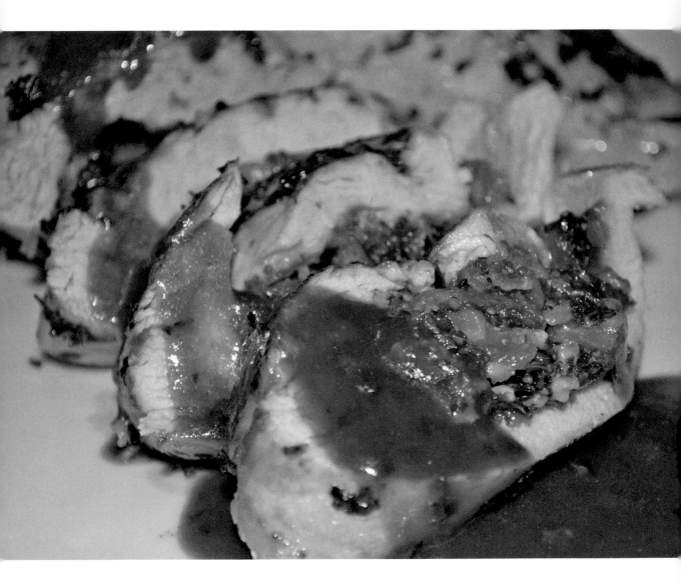

Herb-Crusted Turkey Breast Stuffed with Shallots and Figs NS

1. Preheat oven to 350 degrees.

2. Finely chop fresh herbs. Place in a small bowl, and set aside.

3. Heat 2 teaspoons olive oil and 1 teaspoon ghee in a skillet over medium heat. Sauté shallots for 2 to 3 minutes. Add figs and kale, and sauté an additional 4 to 5 minutes. Remove from heat, and toss with cheese.

4. Slice turkey breast in half to create two pieces. Butterfly each turkey breast by placing on a cutting board and carefully slicing horizontally through the meat, but not all the way to the other side. This opens the breast so that stuffing it is made simple. Spoon half the kale stuffing into each turkey breast. Gently pull the turkey back together, and fasten with toothpicks. Sprinkle both sides of the stuffed turkey breasts with reserved herb mixture.

5. Heat remaining olive oil in an oven-safe skillet over medium heat. Sear stuffed turkey breasts, 3 to 4 minutes per side. Place skillet in oven and cook for 8 to 10 minutes, or until juices run clear and the internal temperature of the turkey reaches 165 degrees.

6. Remove turkey from pan and set on a cutting board to rest. In the meantime, place the baking dish on the burner over medium heat and add remaining ghee and flour, whisking into a paste. Slowly add stock, whisking continuously to form a gravy. Bring to a simmer and cook 2 to 3 minutes, until the gravy coats the back of a spoon.

7. Slice turkey breast, and drizzle with gravy.

*See Vegetable Stock NS recipe (page 210).

▶ SERVES 4

1 tablespoon fresh oregano

2 tablespoons fresh thyme

2 tablespoons fresh basil

1 tablespoon olive oil, divided

1 teaspoon plus 1 tablespoon ghee, divided

½ cup shallots, minced

¾ cup chopped figs (fresh or dried)

2 cups chopped kale

½ cup soft goat cheese

1 large, boneless turkey breast

1 tablespoon brown rice flour

1 cup turkey or Vegetable Stock*

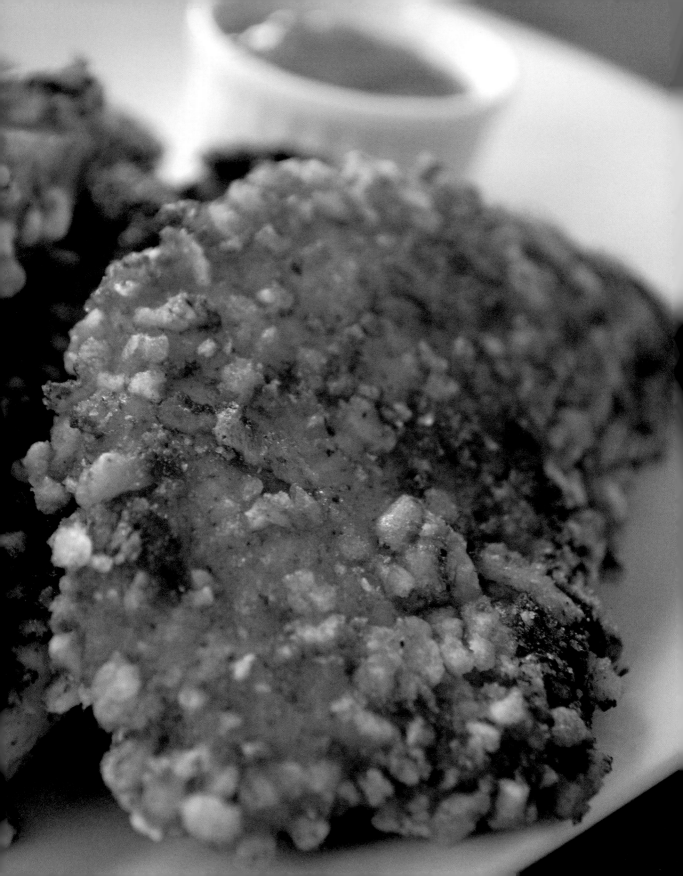

Crispy-Coated Turkey Tenders with Apricot Dipping Sauce (NS)

1. Grind rice cakes in a food processor or mini chopper until they are small crumbs. Pour in a shallow bowl, and add paprika and salt. Toss to combine.

2. In another shallow bowl, whisk egg and almond milk. Dip tenderloins in egg mixture and then into the rice-cake mixture to coat each side.

3. Preheat oven to 375 degrees. Grease a baking sheet with non-stick spray, and set aside.

4. Heat olive oil in a large, oven-safe skillet over medium heat. Brown tenderloins, about 5 minutes per side. Place onto prepared baking sheet and bake 8 minutes or until the internal temperature reaches 165 degrees.

5. While the turkey cooks, combine all dipping sauce ingredients. Mix well.

6. Serve warm.

▶ SERVES 4

tip: If you do not have an oven-safe skillet, simply wrap plastic handle with tinfoil.

2 rice cakes

1 teaspoon sweet paprika

½ teaspoon sea salt

1 large egg

2 teaspoons almond milk

4 turkey tenderloins

1 tablespoon olive oil

Nonstick cooking spray

dipping sauce:

2 teaspoons dry mustard

2 tablespoons (no sugar added) apricot spread

1 teaspoon lemon juice

Turkey Sausage–Zucchini Boats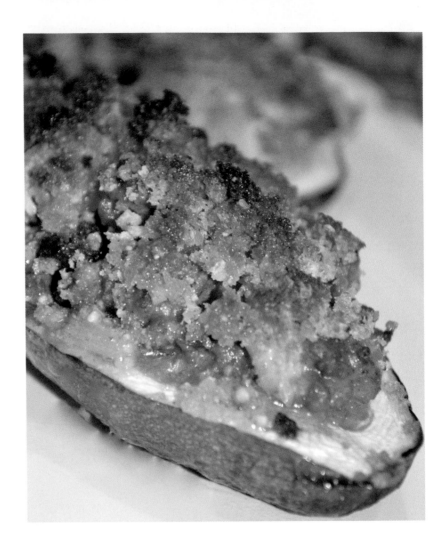

NS

4 large zucchini

2 tablespoons olive oil, divided

1 teaspoon fennel seeds

2 cloves garlic

¼ teaspoon mustard powder

1 cup diced onion

1 fennel bulb, diced

1 pound lean ground turkey

1 tablespoon fresh thyme

2 tablespoons oat flour

1¼ cups chicken broth

1 (6½-oz.) can pimiento

1 cup bread crumbs*

1. Preheat oven to 400 degrees.

2. Slice zucchini in half lengthwise. Use a spoon to scoop out the seeds, trying not to dig too deep into the flesh of the zucchini. Set zucchini skin side down on a baking sheet, drizzle with 2 teaspoons olive oil, and bake for 20 minutes.

3. In a medium skillet, heat olive oil over medium heat. Cook fennel seeds, garlic, and mustard powder in remaining olive oil for 1 minute, just to bring out the flavors. Add onion and fennel, and sauté for 4 minutes. Add ground turkey, breaking large pieces apart with a flat wooden spoon.

4. Once turkey is crumbled, add thyme and sprinkle with flour, tossing to coat. Slowly pour chicken broth over the turkey mixture, stirring constantly, to create a sauce. Bring the sauce to a simmer, then reduce heat to low.

5. Puree pimiento in a mini chopper and add to skillet. Cook 5 to 6 minutes, or until turkey is cooked through.

6. Remove zucchini from the oven. Spoon turkey mixture evenly into each roasted zucchini half, top with bread crumbs, and drizzle 1 teaspoon olive oil over each. Place zucchini back into the oven, and bake 12 minutes or until steaming hot and bread crumbs are golden brown.

*See Basic Bread crumbs NS recipe (page 210).

▶ SERVES 6

Shredded Turkey Bake NS

3 teaspoons olive oil, divided

1 cup diced carrots

1 cup diced onion

2 tablespoons plus 1 teaspoon fresh thyme, divided

2 cups carrot juice

1 cup Vegetable Stock*

⅛ teaspoon sea salt, plus additional, to taste

1½ pounds turkey tenderloin

1 tablespoon arrowroot starch

2 tablespoons cold water

½ cup quinoa

1 cup quartered asparagus spears

1½ cups bread crumbs*

½ cup shredded mozzarella cheese

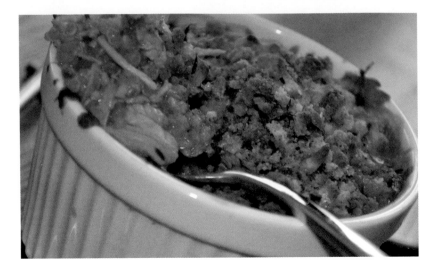

1. Heat 2 teaspoons olive oil in a Dutch oven over medium heat. Add carrots and onion, and sauté for 5 minutes. Add 2 tablespoons thyme, carrot juice, stock, and salt, and stir just to combine. Add turkey tenderloin. Bring mixture to a boil, cover, reduce heat to low, and simmer.

2. After 1½ hours, remove turkey, and shred into bite-size pieces. Return to the pot and increase heat to medium, letting the carrot juice reduce. In a small bowl, dissolve arrowroot starch in water. Add to shredded turkey mixture and cook 10 minutes, until sauce is thickened. Add quinoa and asparagus spears, cook an additional 12 minutes.

3. Mix bread crumbs with remaining 1 teaspoon olive oil, ⅛ teaspoon salt, and the remaining 1 teaspoon fresh thyme. Toss with cheese.

4. Spoon turkey mixture into 6 (7-oz.) individual ramekins, top with bread-crumb mixture, and bake for 8 to 10 minutes or until turkey mixture is bubbling and topping is melted.

▶ SERVES 6

*See Vegetable Stock NS recipe (page 210). See Basic Bread Crumbs NS recipe (page 210).

1. Heat olive oil in a large stockpot over medium heat. Sauté onion and garlic for 4 to 5 minutes. Remove from heat and set aside.

2. Add turkey and break apart with a flat spatula to crumble into small pieces. Cook until brown and cooked through, approximately 5 minutes.

3. Puree spinach in a food processor or blender with stock to create a smooth sauce.

4. Add spinach mixture and remaining ingredients to stockpot. Cover and let simmer at least 45 minutes. Stir occasionally to prevent burning.

5. Serve warm.

*See Vegetable Stock NS recipe (page 210).

▶ SERVES 4

2 teaspoons olive oil

2 cups yellow onion

2 cloves garlic, minced

1 pound ground organic turkey

6 cups spinach

½ cup Vegetable Stock*

1½ cups frozen artichoke hearts, thawed and diced

¼ teaspoon cinnamon

2 teaspoons sweet paprika

1 teaspoon cumin

1 can adzuki beans

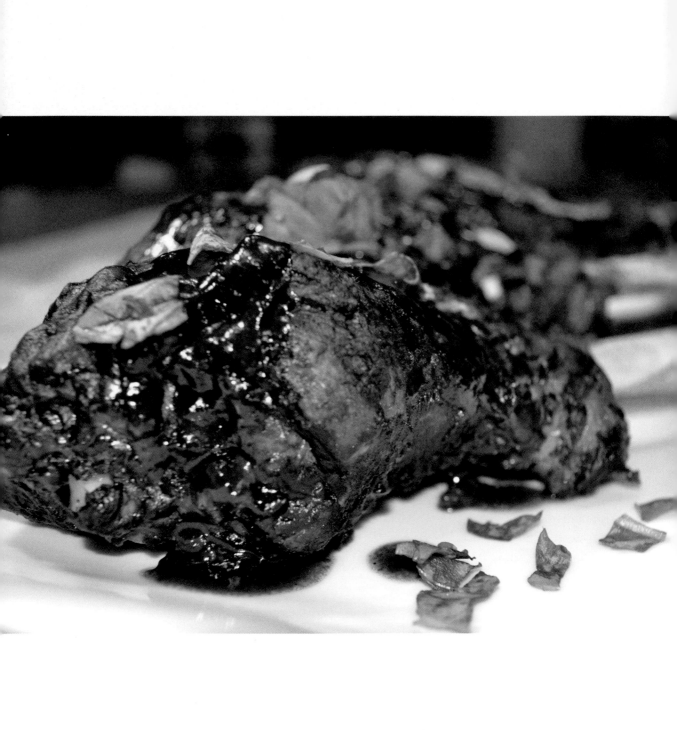

Turkey Mole Drumsticks
NS

1. Preheat oven to 325 degrees.

2. Heat ghee in a medium skillet over medium heat. Sauté garlic and onion for 4 to 5 minutes, until tender and slightly browned. Add seasonings. Stir to combine and cook an additional 2 minutes. Add stock and peanut butter. Stir to combine and cook 3 to 4 minutes.

3. Remove from heat, stir in chocolate, and transfer to a food processor. Puree until smooth. As an optional step, push mole sauce through a strainer to have a silky-smooth sauce.

4. Remove skin from turkey drumsticks, and coat with mole sauce, reserving 2 tablespoons of sauce for later. Place in a baking dish, cover, and bake for 1 to 1 ½ hours. Check internal temperature until it reaches 165 degrees.

5. Once cooked, remove from oven, and serve warm. Top with reserved mole sauce.

*See Vegetable Stock NS recipe (page 210)

*Chicken drumsticks can be used in this recipe, but preheat oven to 400 degrees and bake for 50 to 55 minutes. Juices should run clear and internal temperature should also reach 165 degrees.

▶ SERVES 2

1 teaspoon ghee

2 cloves garlic, minced

¼ cup diced onion

1 teaspoon cumin

1 teaspoon sea salt

1 teaspoon paprika

½ teaspoon cinnamon

1 cup Vegetable Stock*

2 teaspoons peanut butter

1 ounce 100 percent dark chocolate, shaved

3 turkey drumsticks*

 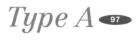

Shepherd's Pie Topped with Roasted Garlic– Whipped Cauliflower 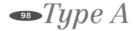 NS

2½ teaspoons olive oil, divided

3 cloves garlic, divided

Sea salt, to taste

1 head cauliflower

1 tablespoon chopped fresh sage

1 tablespoon ghee, divided

6 tablespoons soy or goat milk

Sea salt, to taste

1 pound lean, ground organic turkey

2 teaspoons paprika

2 tablespoons spelt or oat flour

1½ cups Vegetable Stock*

2 cups pearl onions*

1 cup peas

2 cups finely diced carrots

1 cup mozzarella cheese

1. Preheat oven to 375 degrees.

2. Drizzle ½ teaspoon olive oil over two cloves of garlic and season with sea salt. Wrap garlic in parchment paper and then tinfoil, so the foil is fully covering the seasoned garlic. Roast for 30 minutes. Remove from oven and set aside.

3. Reduce oven temperature to 350 degrees.

4. Dice cauliflower into bite-size pieces. Place in a large stockpot full of water and bring to a boil. Cook for 12 to 15 minutes, or just until tender. Drain and place back into the emptied pot. Using a hand mixer, beat cauliflower with roasted garlic, sage, ghee, and milk. Season with sea salt, to taste.

5. Heat remaining 2 teaspoons olive oil in a large skillet over medium heat. Add ground turkey, and break into bits using a flat-ended spatula. Brown for 5 minutes. Add paprika and flour, stirring to coat. Add stock, and bring to a simmer. Reduce the heat, and let cook for 5 minutes, until sauce is thickened.

6. Add onions, peas, and carrots to the turkey and stir to combine. Pour into a large 9" x 11" baking dish, top with cauliflower mixture, spreading evenly across the top with an offset spatula. Sprinkle on cheese and bake for 30 to 35 minutes, until bubbling and cheese is slightly browned.

7. Serve warm.

*See Vegetable Stock recipe NS (page 210).

▶ SERVES 6

*Frozen pearl onions can be used in this recipe instead of fresh as a time saver.

Hearty Slow-Cooker Turkey Stew NS

1. Preheat slow cooker to medium.

2. Heat olive oil in a large skillet over medium heat. Brown turkey breast on all sides, about 1 minute per side . Remove from the pan and set aside.

3. Add onion and parsnips, and sauté 3 to 4 minutes. Remove from skillet and transfer to slow cooker. Add rosemary and thyme. Place turkey breast on top of vegetables and herbs.

4. Combine water and stock in the bottom of the skillet to deglaze and heat for 8 to 10 minutes over medium heat, scraping up all the bits. Pour liquid over turkey and cover.

4. Let cook 1 hour. Add the kale and cook 1 additional hour.

5. Serve warm.

*See Vegetable Stock NS recipe (page 210).

▶ SERVES 4

2 teaspoons olive oil

1 pound turkey breast

2 cups diced onion

2 cups diced parsnips

2 large sprigs fresh rosemary

4 large sprigs fresh thyme

1 cup water

1 cup Vegetable Stock*

4 cups red kale, torn

Red Quinoa– Mushroom Casserole NS

1 cup red quinoa

2 cups water

2 teaspoons ghee

1 cup diced maitake mushrooms

1½ cups diced okra

½ cup finely diced shallots

½ teaspoon mustard powder

½ teaspoon dry ginger

2 cloves garlic, minced

2 tablespoons fresh oregano

¾ cup finely diced pineapple

½ cup diced enoki mushrooms

1 cup Vegetable Stock*

5 eggs, divided

1 teaspoon olive oil

Nonstick olive oil spray

1. Preheat oven to 350 degrees. Grease a 9" x 11" baking dish with olive oil and set aside.

2. Bring quinoa and water to a boil in a medium saucepan. Reduce heat and simmer for 12 minutes. Remove from heat, and fluff with a fork.

3. Melt ghee in large skillet over medium heat. Add maitake mushrooms, okra, and shallots, and sauté 6 to 7 minutes, until vegetables are slightly tender.

4. In a small bowl, whisk mustard powder, ginger, garlic, oregano, pineapple, enoki mushrooms, stock, and 1 egg. Toss quinoa with mushroom mixture, and place into prepared baking dish. Pour broth mixture evenly over casserole. Use a fork to make sure the liquid reaches all corners of the casserole.

5. Bake for 35 minutes.

6. Just before removing casserole, fry remaining eggs in olive oil in a skillet, and serve on top of casserole.

7. Serve warm.

*See Vegetable Stock recipe NS (page 210).

▶ SERVES 6

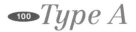

featured ingredient

red quinoa

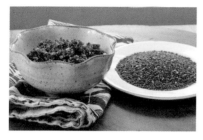

Red quinoa is almost identical in nutritional content to regular quinoa, and it is a terrific source of fiber and protein, as it contains all nine essential amino acids. It also has a similar texture: light and fluffy with a slight crunch. The difference is that red quinoa has an earthier and less bitter taste. Use red quinoa in savory recipes, adding hearty vegetables, allowable cheeses, or beans.

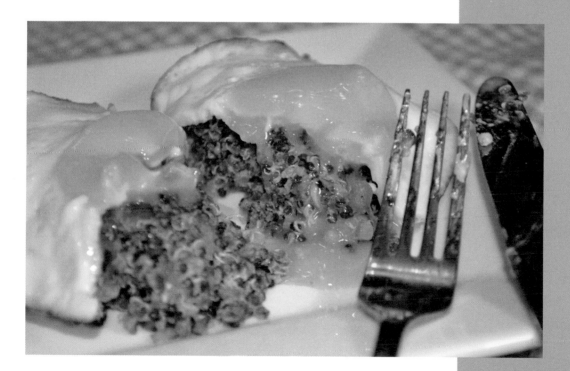

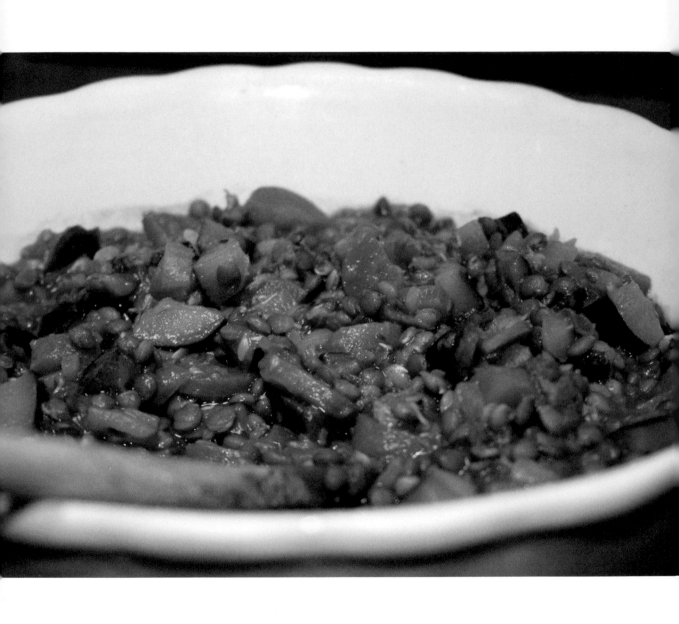

1. Soak sprouted lentils in warm water for 25 minutes.

2. In a large Dutch oven set over to medium heat, add olive oil, onions, carrots, parsnips, zucchini, and cumin. Sauté 6 to 7 minutes. Add lentils and cook 1 additional minute.

3. Add stock one cup at a time, stirring after each addition. Season with salt, to taste. Cook a total of 30 to 35 minutes.

4. Serve warm.

*See Vegetable Stock recipe NS (page 210).

▶ SERVES 4

1 cup sprouted lentils
1 tablespoon olive oil
1 cup diced onions
¾ cup diced carrots
¾ cup diced parsnips
2 zucchini, diced
½ teaspoon cumin
5 cups Vegetable Stock*
Sea salt, to taste

featured ingredient

sprouted lentils

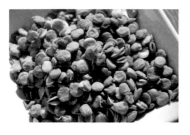

Anytime you see the word *sprouted* in connection with a grain, legumes, or seeds it simply means that the food enzymes have been activated. This results in an increased nutrient content of the grains, legumes, or seeds. Sprouted lentils can be found at most natural food stores, and cook up much faster than lentils that have not been sprouted, so it is a great addition to your "fast food" repertoire!

 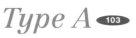

Rice and Bean Loaf

NS

½ cup brown rice, uncooked

1 cup water

2 cups shredded zucchini

½ cup diced onions

½ cup diced carrots

1 large egg, lightly beaten

2 cloves garlic, minced

½ cup bread crumbs*

¾ cup adzuki beans, drained and rinsed

1 teaspoon paprika

½ cup cannellini beans, pureed

Nonstick cooking spray

1. Preheat oven to 350 degrees. Grease an 8½" x 4½" loaf pan with nonstick cooking spray and set aside.

2. Cook rice with water according to package instructions. Let cool.

3. After shredding zucchini, spoon onto a double layer of paper towels or cheesecloth, and squeeze out excess liquid. Add zucchini to a large bowl with onion, carrots, rice, egg, garlic, bread crumbs, adzuki beans, and paprika. Toss to evenly distribute ingredients. Lastly, add pureed cannellini beans, stirring again to combine.

4. Pour mixture into prepared pan. Use an offset spatula to spread mixture evenly across the loaf pan and bake 25 to 30 minutes, until loaf becomes firm, warmed through, and slightly browned around the edges.

5. Serve warm.

*See Basic Bread Crumbs NS recipe (page 210).

▶ SERVES 6

1. Remove tofu from packaging and pat dry with a paper towel. Slice tofu in to 6 thick pieces and place on another paper towel to dry each side.

2. In a large wok (or sauté pan), heat 2 teaspoons olive oil over medium heat. Add ginger and sauté 1 minute. Add tofu and stir-fry until browned, about 3 to 4 minutes. Remove from wok and set aside.

3. Add remaining 1 teaspoon olive oil, snow peas, bok choy, and bamboo. Stir-fry 3 to 4 minutes. Add tofu back to the wok along with remaining ingredients. Toss to coat and cook 2 additional minutes.

4. Serve hot.

▶ SERVES 4

8 ounces extra-firm tofu, sliced

3 teaspoons olive oil, divided

2-inch piece ginger, thinly sliced

2 cups snow peas

1 cup sliced bok choy

¼ cup bamboo shoots

⅓ cup plum jam

1 tablespoon lemon juice

1 tablespoon lemon zest

1 tablespoon low sodium soy sauce (made from soy and wheat-free)

1 tablespoon agave

tip: Bamboo shoots are most commonly found in cans, in the ethnic aisle at the grocery store or natural food market. Rinse bamboo shoots and pat dry so they are ready for cooking.

Tangy Pineapple and Tempeh Kabobs NS

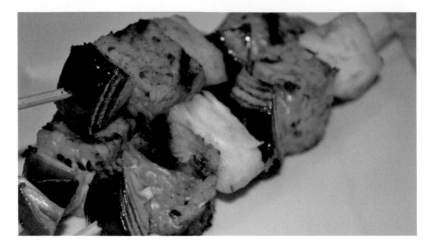

marinade:

2 tablespoons fresh lemon juice

1 tablespoon agave

3 tablespoons olive oil

1 tablespoon minced fresh ginger

½ teaspoon sweet paprika

1 teaspoon garlic, minced

1 (8-oz) package organic flax tempeh

4 cups pineapple pieces

1 red onion, cut into ½-inch dice

1. Whisk all marinade ingredients in a bowl. Dice tempeh into 1–1½-inch cubes. Place diced tempeh in a sealable glass dish and pour two-thirds of the marinade over top. Gently toss to make sure each piece is fully coated with the marinade. Cover and place in the refrigerator for 3 hours.

2. If using bamboo skewers, soak in water for 1 hour to make sure they do not burn during grilling. Alternate one piece of tempeh, pineapple, and onion per skewer. Repeat. Brush pineapple and onion with reserved marinade. Grill for about 10 minutes, flipping halfway through cooking and brushing with any remaining marinade. Tempeh and vegetables should be heated through and have charred grill marks when done.

3. Serve warm.

▶ SERVES 4

featured ingredient

tempeh

Tempeh is fermented soybeans that are pressed into a ½-inch to 1-inch cake, providing a firm texture and slightly nutty taste. Popular in Indonesia, tempeh has become popular among vegetarians in the United States. Like tofu, tempeh has the ability to absorb any flavor you choose to season it with, so it is a perfect canvas for your culinary genius! As a bonus, it is packed with protein and few calories, making it an ideal substitution for beef or other animal protein.

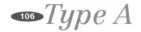

EAT RIGHT FOR YOUR TYPE PERSONALIZED COOKBOOK

Moroccan Tofu Tagine NS

1. Remove tofu from package and slice into ½-inch pieces. Drain on several sheets of paper towel and gently pat excess water from all sides of the tofu pieces.

2. In a small bowl, combine garlic, ginger, cinnamon, cumin, turmeric, and 1 tablespoon olive oil. Gently toss spices with tofu pieces, so as not to break the tofu apart. Marinate in the refrigerator for at least 1 hour.

3. Heat tagine over medium-high and brush with 2 teaspoons olive oil. Sear tofu just until browned on both sides. Remove from tagine and set aside.

4. To the tagine, add remaining 1 teaspoon olive oil, onion, carrots, and parsnips, and cook 5 to 6 minutes.

5. Reduce heat to low. Add stock and lemon juice. Cover tagine and let cook for 30 minutes (and no peeking). At this point, most of the liquid should be absorbed. Return tofu back to tagine, cover, and cook for an additional 10 minutes.

6. Serve warm.

*See Vegetable Stock recipe NS (page 210).

▶ SERVES 4

1 (14-oz.) package firm tofu

2 teaspoons minced garlic

2 teaspoons minced ginger

¼ teaspoon cinnamon

¼ teaspoon cumin

½ teaspoon turmeric

3 teaspoons olive oil, divided

10 cipollini onions

1 cup chopped carrots

1 cup chopped parsnips

½ cup Vegetable Stock*

1 tablespoon lemon juice

tip: A tagine is a Moroccan cooking vessel that has a heavy, cast-iron or clay base and a domed, pyramid-shaped top, which creates a slow cooking method that adds moisture to each dish. As an alternative, try a cast-iron skillet and cover with tented tinfoil. Just make sure to seal the top of the skillet.

 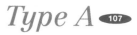

Broccolini-Stuffed Tofu NS

12 ounces extra-firm tofu

1 tablespoon oregano

1 tablespoon lemon juice

1 tablespoon olive oil

Sea salt, to taste

2 teaspoons ghee

1 bunch broccolini, roughly chopped

½ red onion, diced

¼ cup walnuts

⅓ cup crumbled feta cheese

1 cup Vegetable Stock*, divided

1. Slice tofu crosswise into ½-inch-thick squares. Whisk oregano, lemon juice, and olive oil with sea salt. Pour over tofu in an airtight glass container, and let marinate for 30 minutes, flipping once halfway through.

2. In a large skillet, heat ghee over medium heat. Sauté broccolini and onions just until slightly tender, about 2 to 3 minutes. Season with salt, to taste.

3. In a food processor, pulse broccolini and onions with walnuts, cheese, and ¼ cup stock. Filling should be thick and pasty but not too dry. Add more stock if mixture looks dry. Return mixture to skillet over low heat, and keep warm.

4. Remove tofu from marinade and sear in a skillet over medium heat. Cook 1 to 2 minutes or until browned. Turn and brown opposite side, an additional 1 to 2 minutes.

5. To assemble, make 3 layers of tofu topped with broccolini stuffing and serve immediately.

*See Vegetable Stock recipe NS (page 210).

▶ SERVES 4

EAT RIGHT FOR YOUR TYPE PERSONALIZED COOKBOOK

Slow-Cooker Butternut Squash– Lentil Stew NS

1. Turn slow cooker to high.

2. Add all ingredients to the slow cooker. Stir gently to evenly distribute spices and vegetables.

3. Cook 2½ to 3 hours.

4. Serve warm.

*See Vegetable Stock recipe NS (page 210).

▶ SERVES 6

1 cup chopped onion

1 cup chopped carrots

1 tablespoon olive oil, divided

1 pound green lentils

1 teaspoon sea salt

2 cups Vegetable Stock*

2 cups cubed butternut squash

¼ teaspoon cumin

1 teaspoon ground ginger

1 teaspoon garlic powder

¼ teaspoon cinnamon

1 tablespoon chopped fresh sage

3 cups water

 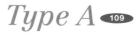

Bean Burgers (NS)

2 cups cooked pinto beans, divided

1½ cups spinach

½ cup carrot, shredded

1 tablespoon olive oil

1 tablespoon fresh thyme

½ teaspoon sea salt

2 cloves garlic, minced

½ cup bread crumbs*

1 large egg, beaten

2 teaspoons olive oil

1. Put 1 cup of beans in a bowl, and smash using a fork or potato masher.

2. In a large bowl, add mashed beans and all remaining ingredients, mixing gently just to combine. Form into 6 patties, and set aside.

3. Heat a large skillet over medium, and drizzle with olive oil. Cook the bean burgers about 4 minutes per side.

4. Serve warm. Delicious with caramelized onions, toasted sprouted wheat rolls, and crunchy lettuce.

*See Basic Bread Crumbs NS recipe (page 210).

▶ SERVES 4

Soups and Sides

Thai Curry Soup NS ■ *Carrot-Ginger Soup* NS ■ *Roasted Parsnip Soup* NS ■ *Melted Mozzarella–Onion Soup* NS ■ *Broccoli–Northern Bean Soup* NS ■ *Tofu and Shredded Escarole Soup* NS ■ *Wild-Grain Soup with Basil Pesto* NS ■ *Crunchy Kohlrabi Slaw* NS ■ *Grilled Sesame-Ginger Bok Choy* NS ■ *Sweet-and-Salty Brussels* NS ■ *South Indian–Curried Okra* NS ■ *Baked Beans* NS ■ *Bacon and Bean Collards* NS ■ *Garlic-Creamed Artichoke Spinach* NS ■ *Roasted Autumn Roots* NS ■ *Roasted Broccoli with Garlic-Basil Oil* NS ■ *Roasted Chestnuts and Rice* NS ■ *Roasted Pumpkin with Fried Sage* NS ■ *Kohlrabi Gratin with Sage-Walnut Cream* NS ■ *Ratatouille* NS ■ *Whipped Pumpkin Soufflé* NS ■ *Rutabaga Smash* NS ■ *Fennel Hash with Turkey Sausage* NS ■ *Pumpkin Ragu* NS ■ *Brown Rice Salad* NS ■ *Forbidden Black Rice Risotto* NS ■ *Herbed Quinoa* NS ■ *Crisp-Tender Veggie Quinoa* ■ *Mint and Pumpkin Tabbouleh* NS ■ *Roasted Escarole* NS ■ *Creamy Rice Polenta* NS

Many times when preparing dinner, we think about eating a protein, vegetable, and complex carbohydrate, and although having them all together in one pot like chili or lasagna is ideal, it doesn't always work out that way. Therefore, it is essential to have a collection of quick, delicious, side or soup options to pair up with your protein choice. In this section, you'll find a number of vegetable-based or complex carbohydrate–based soups and sides to keep on hand.

Thai Curry Soup (NS)

2–3 teaspoons olive oil

1 cup diced leeks

1 teaspoon garlic, minced

1 tablespoon ginger, minced

⅛ teaspoon turmeric

½ teaspoon curry powder

2 small turnips, diced

4 cups water

1 lemongrass stick

3 cups julienned Swiss chard

Sea salt, to taste

cream sauce:

3 tablespoons chopped walnuts

2 tablespoons almond flour (see tip)

1 teaspoon agave

3 tablespoons hot water or almond milk

1. Heat olive oil in a stockpot over medium heat. Sauté leeks, garlic, and ginger for 3 to 4 minutes, until slightly tender and aromatic. Add turmeric, curry powder, and turnips. Stir and cook 5 minutes.

2. Prepare lemongrass by cutting off the white, woody base, and then bruising the stem with the back of a knife. This will help bring out the flavors of the lemongrass. Pour water over vegetables, and add bruised lemongrass, and Swiss chard. Cover, and let simmer at least 30 minutes. Season with sea salt to taste.

3. While the soup simmers, place walnuts and almond flour in a food processor or mini chopper. Pulse until nuts become pasty. Gradually drizzle in agave and hot water, and continue to puree until smooth and creamy.

4. Add cream sauce to soup and let cook 5 minutes.

5. Serve warm.

▶ SERVES 6

tip: If you do not have almond flour, pulse ¼ cup raw, blanched almonds in a food processor until finely ground.

featured ingredient

lemongrass

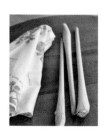

Lemongrass is a thick, woody stalk that needs to be bruised and chopped when used in cooking to help bring out its flavor. Lemongrass is most widely used in Asian cooking and adds a fresh, citrus flavor to dishes. For centuries, lemongrass has been thought to have healing properties.

Carrot-Ginger Soup (NS)

1. In a stockpot, heat olive oil and ghee over medium heat. Add onion, garlic, and carrots, sautéing 5 to 6 minutes until vegetables become tender. Add remaining ingredients, and bring to a boil. Reduce heat to a simmer, cover, and cook at least 30 minutes, or until carrots are fork-tender.

2. Puree soup with an immersion blender or standing blender until smooth. If the mixture appears too thick, add water until desired consistency.

3. Serve warm.

▶ SERVES 6

1 teaspoon olive oil

2 teaspoons ghee

1 cup chopped onion

1 clove garlic

2 pounds carrots, peeled and diced

1 3-inch piece (or about ¼ cup) ginger, peeled and grated

½ teaspoon sea salt

1 tablespoon lemon zest

4 cups water

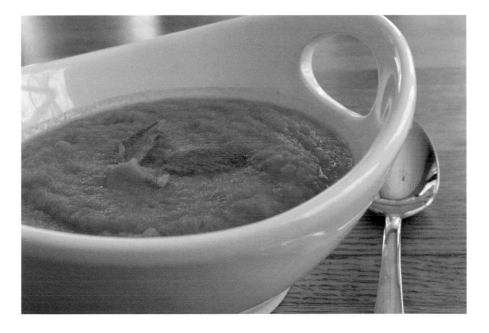

Roasted Parsnip Soup NS

4 cups diced parsnips

4 cups diced cauliflower

2 cloves garlic, peeled

2 tablespoons olive oil, divided

Sea salt, to taste

2 cups finely sliced sweet onion

2 finely diced Granny Smith apples

1½ cups soy or almond milk

1 cup water

⅛ teaspoon nutmeg

¼ cup chopped fresh sage

1. Preheat oven to 375 degrees.

2. Place parsnips, cauliflower, and garlic on a sheet pan, drizzle with 1 tablespoon olive oil and sprinkle with sea salt. Toss to coat.

3. Roast vegetables in the oven for 35 to 40 minutes, or until tender and golden brown around the edges.

4. About 15 minutes before the vegetables are finished cooking, heat remaining 1 tablespoon olive oil in a large stockpot over medium heat. Sauté onion for 8 to 10 minutes. Add apples and sauté an additional 3 to 4 minutes.

5. Once the onions are tender, add roasted vegetables and remaining ingredients to the pot. Bring the soup to a gentle boil and simmer for 20 minutes. Blend with an immersion blender, or puree in a standing blender.

6. Season with additional sea salt, to taste, and serve warm.

▶ SERVES 6

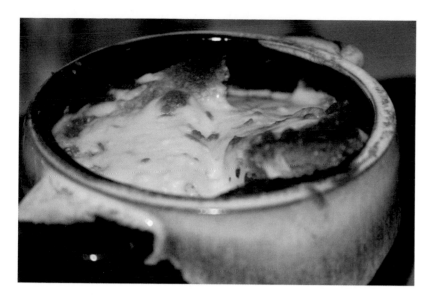

Melted Mozzarella–Onion Soup NS

5 large white onions

1 tablespoon olive oil

½ tablespoon ghee

½ cup red or white wine

3 cups Vegetable Stock*

4 sprigs thyme

2 sprigs sage

2 bay leaves

Sea salt, to taste

4 slices sprouted bread, toasted

1 cup grated mozzarella cheese

1. Peel onions, slice in half, and then slice in thin, half-moon shapes.

2. Heat olive oil and ghee in a large-bottomed stockpot over medium heat. Add onion and caramelize for 12 minutes. Season with sea salt, reduce the cooking temperature to medium-low, and cook an additional 20 minutes. Onions will become a rich, caramel color as the natural sugars in the onions release and sweeten them.

3. Add wine to the onions to deglaze the pan (helping the delicious bits on the bottom of the pan come up and mingle with the onions) and cook another 30 seconds. Add thyme, sage, bay leaves, salt, and broth. Simmer for 30 minutes.

4. Spoon soup into 4 individual (7-oz.) high-sided, oven-safe bowls or ramekins. Place 1 slice of toast on each ramekin, then sprinkle with cheese.

5. Broil in oven for 2 minutes or until the cheese begins to bubble and brown slightly. Keep a close eye, as the toast and cheese can burn quickly.

6. Serve warm.

*See Vegetable Stock recipe NS (page 210).

▶ SERVES 4

Broccoli–Northern Bean Soup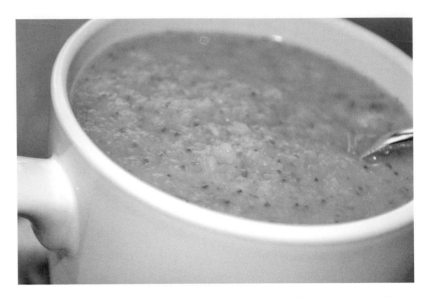

NS

1 tablespoon olive oil, divided

1 cup diced white onion

2 heads broccoli

1 clove garlic, minced

1 (15-oz.) can northern beans (BPA-free can), rinsed and drained

2 cups Vegetable Stock*

4 sprigs fresh thyme

Sea salt, to taste

¼ cup pine nuts

1. Heat 2 teaspoons olive oil in a large stockpot over medium heat. Sauté onions for 5–6 minutes.

2. Trim woody stems off broccoli and discard. Rough chop the broccoli and remaining stems. Add to the onions along with garlic, beans, stock, and thyme. Bring to a boil, and reduce to simmer for 15 minutes. Vegetables should be tender and easily pierced with a fork, but not falling apart.

3. Using an immersion blender or stand blender, puree soup until smooth. Soup should be thick and creamy, but easily run off your spoon. Add water or additional stock if you prefer a thinner consistency. Season with sea salt, to taste.

4. Heat remaining olive oil in a small skillet over medium heat. Toast pine nuts for 2 to 3 minutes, or until golden brown.

5. Serve soup hot, topped with toasted pine nuts.

*See Vegetable Stock NS recipe (page 210).

▶ SERVES 6

EAT RIGHT FOR YOUR TYPE PERSONALIZED COOKBOOK

Tofu and Shredded Escarole Soup NS

1. Heat 1 teaspoon olive oil in a Dutch oven over medium heat. Sauté ginger and garlic for 30 seconds, stirring continuously to prevent burning. Add remaining olive oil, and then toss in tofu. Cook until browned. Remove from pot and set aside.

2. Add stock, water, onion, bay leaf, and carrots. Simmer over medium-low heat for 30 minutes.

3. About 10 minutes before serving, add beans and return tofu to the soup. Spoon into bowls, and top each bowl with ½ cup escarole.

*See Vegetable Stock NS recipe (page 210).

▶ SERVES 4

2 teaspoons olive oil, divided

1-inch piece fresh ginger, minced

1 clove garlic, minced

12 ounces extra-firm tofu, cubed

Sea salt, to taste

2 cups Vegetable Stock*

3 cups water

1 cup pearl onions

1 bay leaf

1 cup carrots, cut into matchsticks

2 cups haricot vert

2 cups shredded escarole

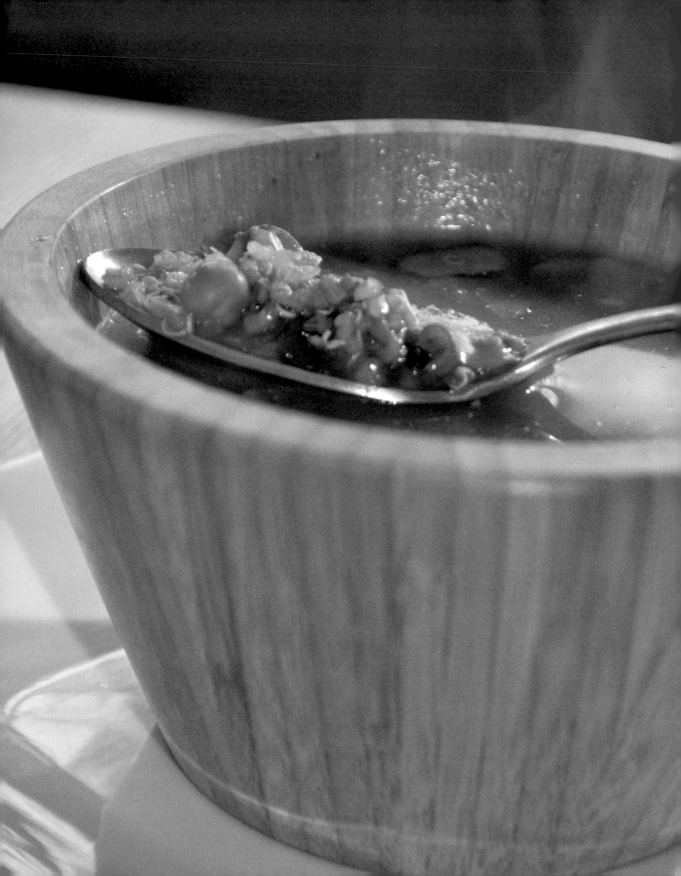

Wild-Grain Soup with Basil Pesto NS

1. Cook rice according to package instructions. Remove from heat and transfer to a bowl to cool.

2. In the same pot, melt ghee over medium heat and add garlic and mushrooms. Sauté 3 to 4 minutes. Add stock and water, and bring to boil. Reduce heat and simmer 5 minutes.

3. Combine peas, basil, garlic, olive oil, lemon juice, walnuts, and water. Season with sea salt, to taste, and set aside.

4. Add raw quinoa to the soup and let simmer an additional 10 minutes. Add snow peas and cook 3 minutes. Serve with a dollop of pesto.

*See Vegetable Stock NS recipe (page 210).

▶ SERVES 6

½ cup wild brown rice
2 teaspoons ghee
1 clove garlic
8 ounces cremini mushrooms
4 cups Vegetable Stock*
3 cups water

basil pesto:
1 cup cooked peas
½ cup fresh basil
1 clove garlic
2 tablespoons olive oil
2 tablespoons lemon juice
¼ cup raw walnuts
3 tablespoons water
Sea salt, to taste
¼ cup quinoa
¾ cup snow peas

Crunchy Kohlrabi Slaw NS

3 tablespoons lemon juice

3 tablespoons olive oil

2 teaspoons dry mustard

1 teaspoon honey or agave

Sea salt, to taste

3 bulbs kohlrabi

2 bunches broccoli stems

½ cup golden raisins

¼ cup chopped parsley

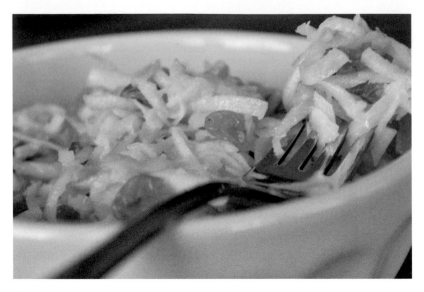

1. Whisk lemon juice, olive oil, mustard, honey, and sea salt, to taste, in the bottom of a large bowl. Set aside.

2. Cut tough bottoms off the kohlrabi as well as stems coming off the top, and peel outer layer. Grate the peeled bulbs into the bowl with the dressing. Cut bottoms and tops off broccoli stems, and peel and grate into the same bowl with kohlrabi. A food processor can also be used for grating.

3. Add raisins and parsley, toss to mix, and coat with dressing. Serve chilled.

▶ SERVES 4

tip: Reserve broccoli and kohlrabi tops for later use. Sauté for 8 to 10 minutes over medium heat with 1 tablespoon olive oil and a dash of sea salt for a delicious side dish any night of the week.

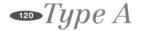

Grilled Sesame-Ginger Bok Choy NS

2 teaspoons olive oil

1 teaspoon soy sauce

1 teaspoon sesame oil

1 tablespoon fresh ginger, grated

1 large bunch of bok choy

1 teaspoon sesame seeds

1. Heat grill pan over medium heat.

2. In a small bowl, whisk together olive oil, soy sauce, sesame oil, and ginger. Set aside.

3. Pull the leaves off the base of the bok choy and slice off the very bottom of the stem to remove any tough pieces. Wash the leaves individually and let them dry completely on a clean kitchen towel.

4. Brush individual bok choy leaves with soy mixture.

5. Grill leaves for about 30 to 45 seconds per side to wilt the bok choy and create grill marks on the stems and leaves.

6. Sprinkle grilled bok choy with sesame seeds and serve warm.

▶ SERVES 4

tip: When purchasing bok choy, look for stalks that are bright white in color with dark-green leaves. Avoid spotted stems and wilted-looking leaves.

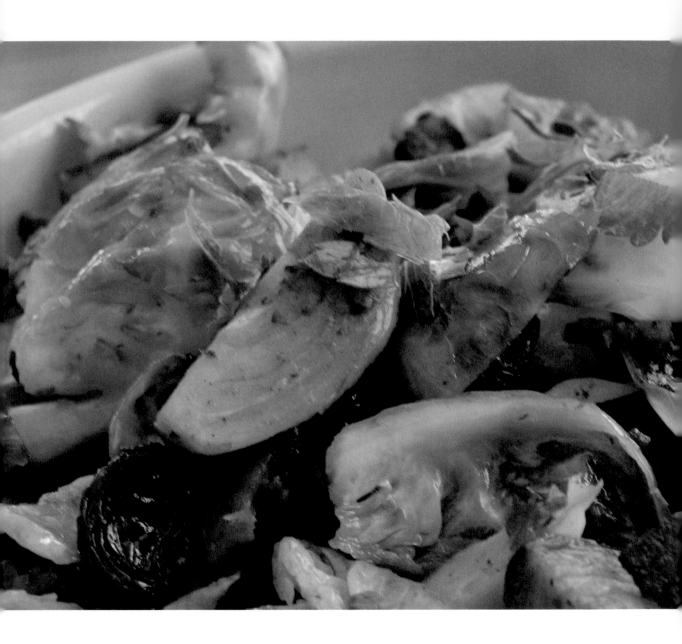

Sweet-and-Salty Brussels NS

1. Heat ghee and olive oil in a large skillet over medium heat. Sauté shallots and turkey bacon until bacon is crispy, about 4 to 5 minutes.

2. Add Brussels sprouts and continue to cook for 15 minutes, stirring occasionally to prevent burning. Add raisins and stock and cook an additional 3 minutes, to allow raisins to become tender and the broth to help deglaze the bottom of the pan and add moisture to the sprouts.

3. Sprouts are done when they can be pierced with a fork but still give moderate resistance. If they are overcooked and become mushy they lose a lot of flavor.

4. Garnish with parsley and serve warm.

*See Vegetable Stock NS recipe (page 210).

▶ SERVES 4

1 teaspoon ghee

2 teaspoons olive oil

2 tablespoons finely diced shallots

4 strips turkey bacon, diced

4 cups quartered Brussels sprouts

¼ cup golden raisins

½ cup Vegetable Stock*

1 tablespoon chopped parsley, for garnish

South Indian–Curried Okra NS

1 tablespoon olive oil

½ teaspoon mustard seeds

½ teaspoon cumin

½ teaspoon urad dal*

¾ cup finely diced onion

3 cups diced okra

4 cups chopped spinach

½ teaspoon turmeric

½ teaspoon sea salt

1. Heat olive oil in a Dutch oven over medium heat. Add mustard seed, cumin, and urad dal, and cook 30 seconds. Add onion and cook 5 minutes.

2. Add okra and cook an additional 15 minutes. Add spinach, turmeric, and salt, and let cook another 5 minutes until okra is tender, and the spinach is wilted.

3. Serve warm.

► SERVES 6

tip: Urad dal means black lentil, a staple of South India dishes.

Baked Beans NS

1. Preheat oven to 375 degrees.

2. Heat olive oil in a Dutch oven over medium heat. Sauté onion and garlic until translucent and tender, about 5 to 7 minutes. Add mustard, molasses, salt, and paprika, and cook 1 additional minute.

3. Add pinto beans and stock. Stir to combine.

4. Cover and bake for 25 minutes. Beans will be heated through, and the sauce will be thick and aromatic.

5. Serve warm.

*See Vegetable Stock NS recipe (page 210).

▶ SERVES 6

2 teaspoons olive oil

1 cup diced yellow onion

1 clove garlic, minced

1 teaspoon dry mustard

1 tablespoon molasses

1 teaspoon salt

1 teaspoon paprika

2 (15-oz.) cans pinto beans, rinsed and drained

⅓ cup Vegetable Stock*

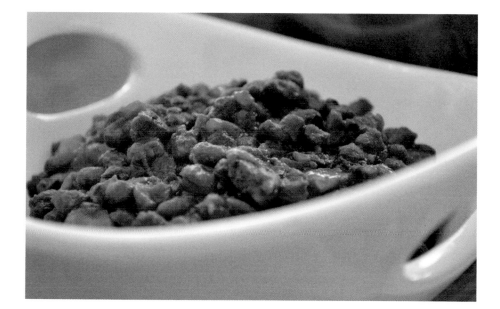

 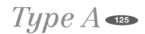

Bacon and Bean Collards NS

2 teaspoons olive oil

1 teaspoon ghee

½ cup diced shallots

4 slices turkey bacon, finely diced

½ teaspoon smoked paprika

1 bunch collard greens

1 (15-oz.) can black-eyed peas, rinsed and drained

Sea salt, to taste

1. Heat olive oil and ghee in large skillet over medium heat. Sauté shallots and bacon for 4 to 5 minutes, until bacon is crispy. Season with paprika, add collard greens, and cook for 10 to 12 minutes. Collards should be tender and wilted.

2. Add black-eyed peas, and cook an additional 3 to 4 minutes, until warmed through.

3. Season with sea salt, and serve warm.

▶ SERVES 4

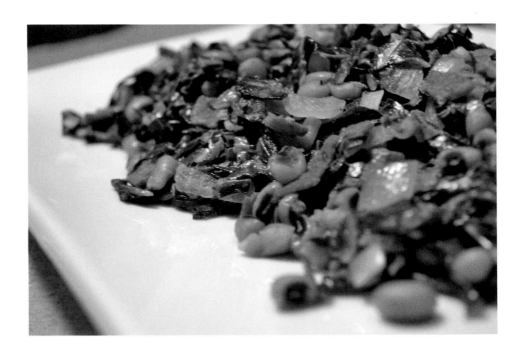

EAT RIGHT FOR YOUR TYPE PERSONALIZED COOKBOOK

Garlic-Creamed Artichoke Spinach NS

1. Heat olive oil in a Dutch oven over medium heat. Sauté garlic, onion, and artichokes for 5 to 6 minutes. Remove vegetables and set aside.

2. In the same pot, melt ghee and add flour. Stir for 1 minute. Slowly add almond milk and stock, whisking continuously to avoid lumps. Continue whisking until mixture becomes the consistency of yogurt, about 5 minutes.

3. Return vegetables to the Dutch oven. Add spinach, one-quarter at a time, just so the spinach has a chance to cook down and make room for the next batch. Season with sea salt to taste.

4. Let cook an additional 5 minutes until spinach wilts, and serve warm.

*See Vegetable Stock NS recipe (page 210).

▶ SERVES 4

2 teaspoons olive oil

2 cloves garlic, minced

1 cup finely diced white onion

1 cup diced frozen artichoke hearts, thawed

1 tablespoon ghee

3 tablespoons spelt flour

½ cup almond milk

¾ cup Vegetable Stock*

Sea salt, to taste

10 cups roughly chopped baby spinach

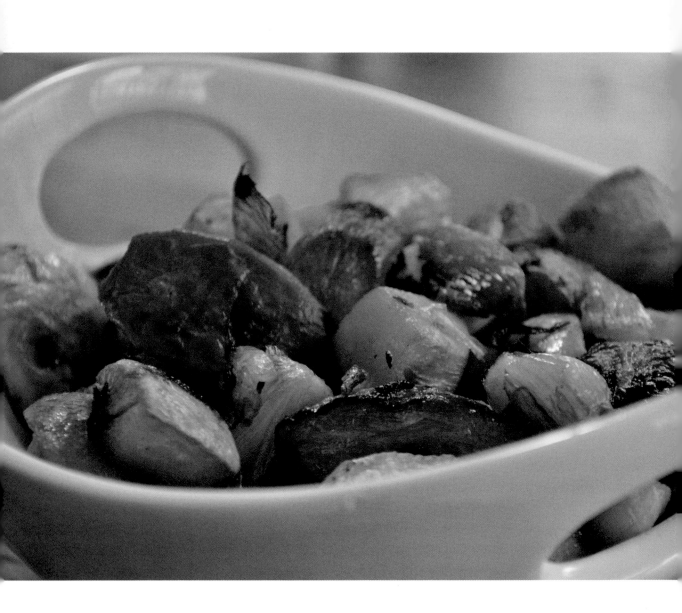

Roasted Autumn Roots NS

1. Preheat oven to 400 degrees.

2. Peel celery root, turnip, pumpkin, and carrots. Dice peeled vegetables into 2-inch pieces.

3. Toss vegetables, shallots, olive oil, sea salt, and sage in a large bowl until evenly coated.

4. Pour onto a baking sheet and bake for 55 to 60 minutes. Vegetables will be browned, crispy on their edges, and soft inside.

5. Serve warm.

▶ SERVES 4

1 celery root

1 turnip

1 small (3-lb.) sugar pumpkin

2 carrots

4 shallots, diced

1 tablespoon olive oil

1 teaspoon sea salt

2 tablespoons fresh chopped sage

featured ingredient

celery root

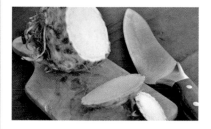

Otherwise known as celeriac, celery root is just what it seems: the root of a type of celery. It has a deliciously fresh flavor that is a cross between celery and parsley, but works terrifically as a base for soups with onions and carrots, eaten raw, or roasted as featured in the Roasted Autumn Roots recipe. A *Neutral* for all blood types, this vegetable adds a diversity of flavor to your palate.

Roasted Broccoli with Garlic-Basil Oil (NS)

1 head broccoli
2 teaspoons olive oil
Sea salt, to taste

basil oil:
1 clove garlic
1 cup finely chopped basil
1 tablespoon lemon juice
1 tablespoon olive oil
1–2 tablespoons water

1. Preheat oven to 375 degrees.

2. Dice broccoli into bite-size pieces and toss with 2 teaspoons olive oil and sea salt. Place on a sheet pan or baking dish and roast for 25 minutes; broccoli will be deep green and slightly browned on the bottom.

3. While the broccoli roasts, puree garlic, basil, lemon juice, olive oil, and water until thin and runny.

4. Serve broccoli drizzled with basil oil.

▶ SERVES 4

Roasted Chestnuts and Rice NS

1. Preheat oven to 400 degrees.

2. Drain chestnuts and let dry on a paper towel. Quarter chestnuts and toss with 2 teaspoons olive oil, sprinkle with ½ teaspoon sea salt, and roast in the oven for 12 minutes. Set aside.

3. Combine stock, water, rice, and remaining ½ teaspoon salt in a 2-quart covered pot. Cook according to package instructions.

4. When rice is finished cooking, fluff with a fork, and toss in apples, chestnuts, and cloves.

5. Serve warm.

*See Vegetable Stock NS recipe (page 210).

▶ SERVES 6

1 cup precooked chestnuts

1 tablespoon olive oil, divided

1 teaspoon sea salt, divided

1 cup Vegetable Stock*

1 cup water

1 cup brown rice

1 cup finely diced Granny Smith apple

⅛ teaspoon ground cloves

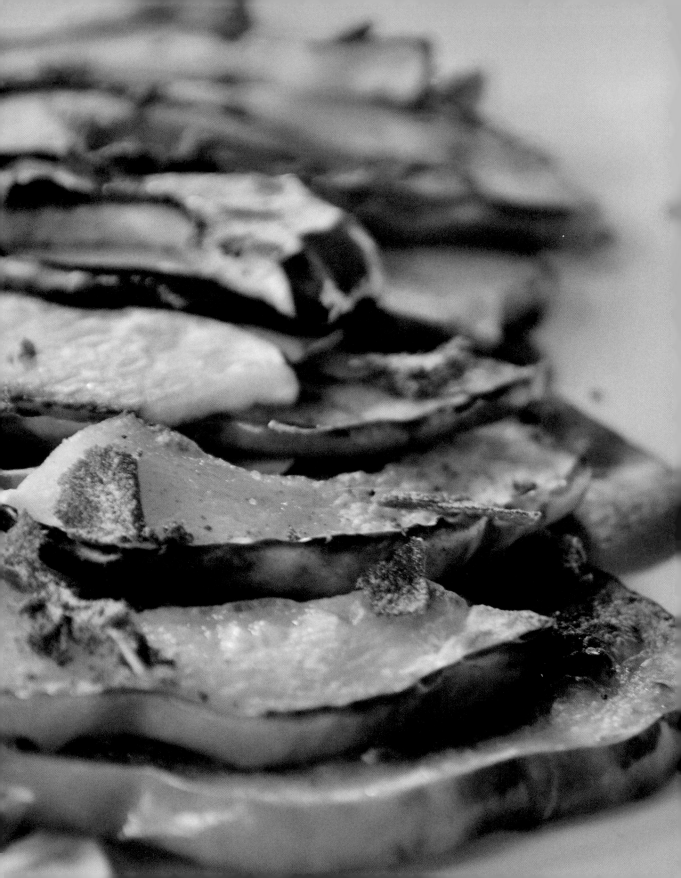

1. Preheat oven to 400 degrees.

2. Very carefully, cut the top off the pumpkin and then slice in half vertically. Use a large metal spoon to remove all seeds and membrane from the pumpkin's cavity. Once cleaned out, turn the pumpkin cut-side down on the cutting board for stability and thinly slice pumpkin into ½-inch sections. Place pumpkin slices in a single layer on a baking sheet, drizzle with 2 teaspoons olive oil, a dash of sea salt, and nutmeg.

3. Roast for 45 to 50 minutes, or until fork-tender.

4. Heat remaining 1 tablespoon olive oil in a small skillet over medium heat. Add sage. Make sure the sage is perfectly dry, as wetness on the leaves will splatter the hot oil. Fry sage until crispy, 30 seconds. Remove with a slotted spoon onto a paper towel.

5. Remove the pumpkin, garnish with crumbled fried sage, and serve immediately.

▶ SERVES 4

1 (4-lb.) sugar pumpkin

1 tablespoon plus 2 teaspoons olive oil

Sea salt, to taste

⅛ teaspoon nutmeg

2 tablespoons fresh sage, dried well

tip: When choosing a pumpkin to roast, opt for a smaller sugar pumpkin, which lends a sweeter flavor. Make sure there are no bruises or weak spots in the flesh and it feels firm. Additionally, the older the pumpkin is, the firmer and more difficult cutting the skin becomes, so the fresher the better.

 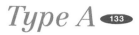

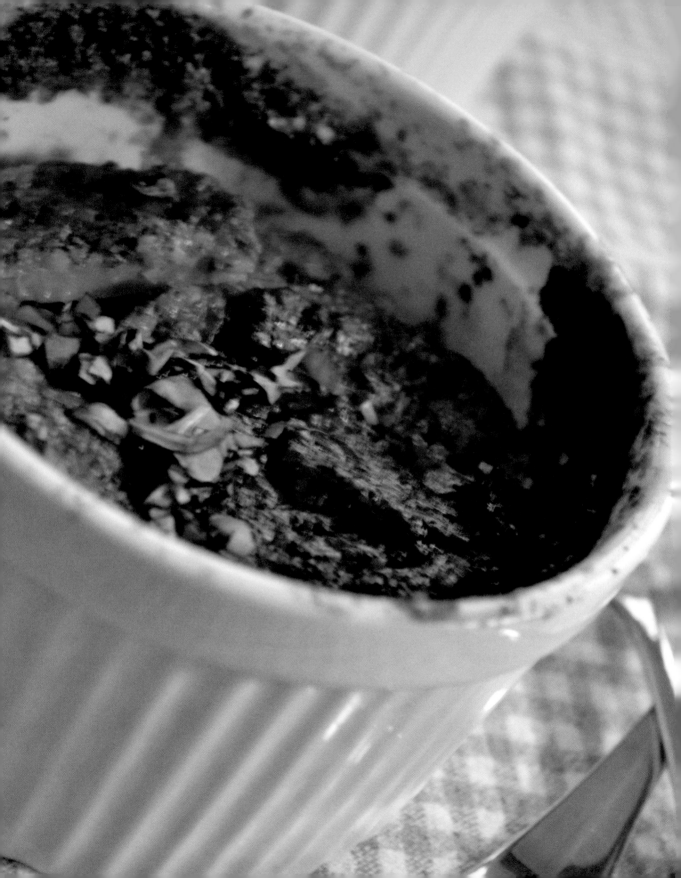

Kohlrabi Gratin with Sage-Walnut Cream NS

2 bulbs kohlrabi

½ cup almond milk

⅛ teaspoon ground cloves

2 tablespoons fresh sage

¼ cup water

½ cup chopped walnuts

Sea salt, to taste

1 cup mozzarella cheese

1. Preheat oven to 375 degrees.

2. Peel kohlrabi, and slice off woody bottom. Place in a pot with enough water to cover by about 1 inch, and boil for 6 to 7 minutes. Drain, slice into ¼-inch rounds, and set aside.

3. In a small saucepan, combine almond milk, cloves, sage, and water and heat until it reaches a boil.
   Reduce to a simmer.

4. In a food processor, pulse walnuts until crumbled. Gradually drizzle in half of the hot milk mixture and puree. Walnut cream should be about the thickness of buttermilk. Add sea salt, to taste.

5. Spoon a small amount of walnut cream in the bottom of 2 (12-oz.) ramekins. Alternate layers of kohlrabi with a spoonful of walnut cream and shredded cheese. Repeat until the layers of kohlrabi have reached the top of the ramekins, and finish with cream and cheese. Pour remaining almond milk evenly over each ramekin, and bake for 30 to 35 minutes. Gratins should be tender and bubbling, and the cheese will be slightly browned and melted.

6. Serve warm.

▶ SERVES 4

Ratatouille

NS

2 medium zucchini

Sea salt, to taste

4 portabella mushrooms

1 bulb fennel

1 cup diced leeks

2 (6½-oz.) jar whole pimientos, drained

1 tablespoon olive oil, divided

½ cup chopped parsley

2 cloves garlic

1. Preheat oven to 375 degrees.

2. Slice zucchini into ¼-inch rounds, set on a towel, and sprinkle with sea salt to draw out excess moisture. Sprinkle salt over the portabella mushrooms, and set on towel. Slice fennel and leeks in a similar fashion, and set aside.

3. Pulse pimientos in a mini food processor a few times until broken up but still chunky.

4. Heat 2 teaspoons olive oil in a large skillet over medium heat. Place fennel, leeks and onion in a single layer in skillet, and cook 2 to 3 minutes per side, just until brown and vegetables begin to cook. Remove from skillet and set aside.

5. Pat excess moisture off zucchini and portabella mushrooms, and brown in the same skillet, cooking 2 to 3 minutes per side, adding additional oil if necessary. Once browned on both sides, remove from pan, and set aside.

6. Finally, sauté pimiento, parsley, and garlic in pan over medium-high heat for 3 to 4 minutes to help some of the liquid from the pimientos evaporate.

7. In a baking dish, layer zucchini and mushrooms across the bottom, top with pimiento mixture, and top with onion and fennel.

8. Bake uncovered for 20 minutes, until bubbling and slightly browned around the edges.

9. Serve warm or at room temperature. Alternatively, store in refrigerator and serve cold.

▶ SERVES 4

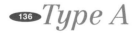

Whipped Pumpkin Soufflé (NS)

1. Preheat oven to 350 degrees. Butter bottoms and sides of 8 (4-oz.) ramekins with ghee, and set aside.

2. In a small saucepan, gently warm 1½ cups milk with 2 sprigs of sage for 10 to 12 minutes.

3. While the milk is heating, whisk egg yolks, brown rice flour, and maple syrup. When milk is ready, temper egg yolks by very slowly pouring about ½ cup of warm milk into the egg mixture, stirring continuously. Pour the tempered eggs back into the saucepan with the remaining milk, and stir over medium heat until thickened, 2 to 3 minutes.

4. In a medium bowl, beat pumpkin with ghee, remaining 1 tablespoon chopped sage, cinnamon, and salt. When milk mixture has thickened, remove from heat and whisk in pumpkin mixture until smooth. Let this mixture cool completely.

5. In a dry glass, stainless steel, or copper bowl, beat egg whites until they form stiff peaks. Fold egg whites into cooled pumpkin mixture, ⅓ at a time. Once the egg whites are completely incorporated, spoon batter into prepared ramekins, filling each ramekin ¾ of the way up the sides. Place ramekins in a high-sided baking dish, and place in oven with the oven rack extended out of the oven. Pour hot water into the bottom of the baking dish to measure 1 inch. Bake soufflés for 55 to 60 minutes or until firm.

6. Serve immediately.

▶ SERVES 6

Ingredients

1½ cups almond, soy, or hemp milk

2 sprigs plus 1 tablespoon fresh sage, chopped

3 egg yolks

¼ cup brown rice flour

1 tablespoon maple syrup

1 cup pumpkin puree

1 tablespoon ghee, softened, plus more for greasing

¼ teaspoon cinnamon

1 teaspoon sea salt

6 large egg whites, whipped

tip: Egg whites cannot be beaten in a bowl that holds fat, such as plastic. Rather, a glass, copper, or stainless steel bowl will enable the eggs to beat into stiff peaks with no problem. Water inside the bowl will also prohibit egg whites from stiffening, so make sure to carefully dry the inside of the bowl before beating.

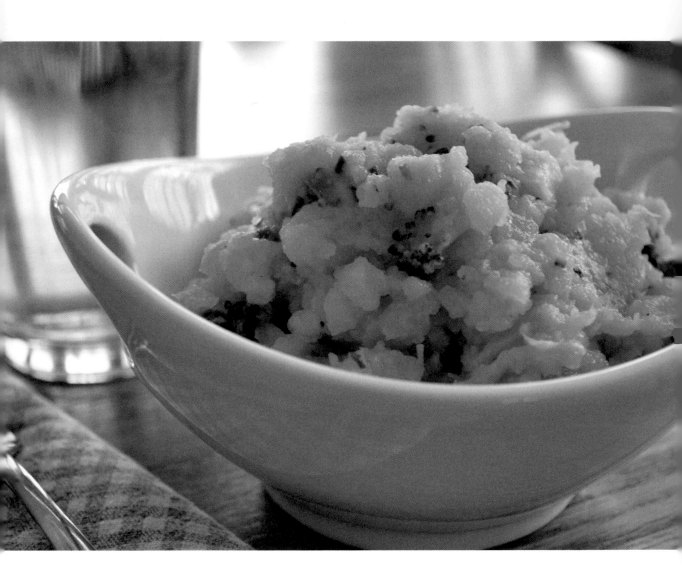

Rutabaga Smash NS

1. Peel rutabaga and dice evenly to ensure even cooking. Place rutabaga in a pot with 2 quarts cold, salted water and bring to a boil. Cover, reduce heat, and simmer for 35 minutes, or until rutabaga is fork-tender.

2. Trim stems off broccoli and dice into bite-size pieces. Steam for 5 to 6 minutes until bright green and slightly tender.

3. When the rutabaga is finished cooking, drain water, and place rutabaga back into the pot on stove. Use a potato masher or fork to mash rutabaga, and add parsley, milk, garlic, ghee, and salt. Cook 3 to 4 minutes until ghee melts and flavors incorporate. Fold broccoli into rutabaga mash.

4. Serve warm.

▶ SERVES 4

2 rutabaga roots
½ teaspoon olive oil
1 head broccoli
¼ cup roughly chopped parsley
¼ cup almond milk
2 cloves garlic, peeled
2 teaspoons ghee
Sea salt, to taste

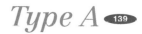

Fennel Hash with Turkey Sausage (NS)

2 teaspoons ghee

2 cups finely sliced onion

3 cups finely sliced fennel

2 links raw turkey sausage, casings removed

2 teaspoons olive oil, as needed

Sea salt, to taste

½ teaspoon cinnamon

1 tablespoon maple syrup

1. In a large skillet, heat ghee over medium heat. Sauté onions and fennel for 3 to 4 minutes. Remove vegetables, and set aside. In the same skillet, add turkey sausage, and break apart with a flat spatula. Add olive oil if needed, and cook until brown and crumbly, 5 to 6 minutes. Season with sea salt to taste.

2. Once sausage is cooked through, add onions, fennel, cinnamon, and maple syrup to the pan, and stir just to combine.

3. Serve hot.

▶ SERVES 4

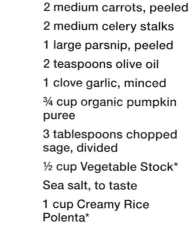

Pumpkin Ragu NS

1. Dice onions, carrots, celery, and parsnips in ¼-inch to ½-inch dice.

2. Heat olive oil in a large sauté pan over medium heat. Add vegetables and sauté 5 to 6 minutes, until vegetables begin to soften.

3. Add garlic, pumpkin, 2 tablespoons sage, and stock, and season with sea salt, to taste. Bring to a bubble, and reduce heat to low. Cook for 20 to 30 minutes, stirring occasionally, until vegetables are fork-tender.

4. Serve warm on top of Creamy Rice Polenta and garnish with remaining sage.

*See Vegetable Stock recipe NS (page 210). See Creamy Rice Polenta NS recipe (page 148).

1 medium onion

2 medium carrots, peeled

2 medium celery stalks

1 large parsnip, peeled

2 teaspoons olive oil

1 clove garlic, minced

¾ cup organic pumpkin puree

3 tablespoons chopped sage, divided

½ cup Vegetable Stock*

Sea salt, to taste

1 cup Creamy Rice Polenta*

▶ SERVES 4

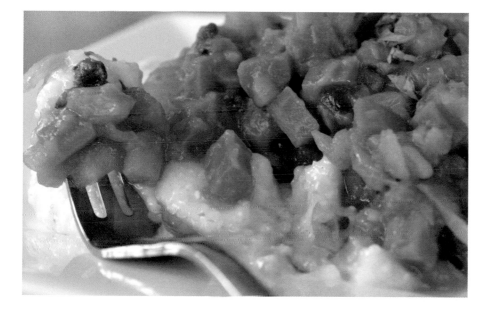

 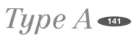

Brown Rice Salad NS

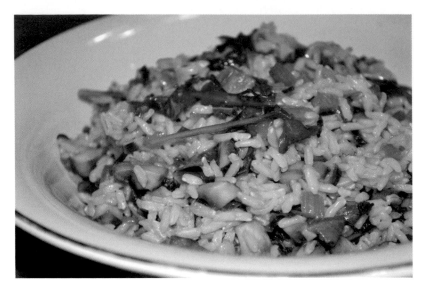

¾ cup brown rice

2 teaspoons olive oil

½ cup diced celery

1 tablespoon sage

2 cups diced cremini mushrooms

¼ cup finely diced shallots

2 cups arugula

2 tablespoons toasted almonds

1. Cook brown rice according to package instructions. Set aside to cool slightly.

2. Heat olive oil in a medium skillet over medium heat. Sauté celery, sage, mushrooms, and shallots for 3 to 4 minutes. Vegetables should just begin to soften.

3. In a large serving bowl, toss brown rice, sautéed mushroom mixture, arugula, and toasted almonds. The warm brown rice will wilt the arugula slightly.

4. Serve warm or room temperature.

▶ SERVES 4

Forbidden Black Rice Risotto NS

1. Heat olive oil in a Dutch oven over medium heat. Sauté onion and rice for 3 to 4 minutes, stirring constantly.

2. In a small pot, heat stock and milk. Slowly add one ladle of the liquid at a time to the rice and onions. When the liquid is absorbed, add the next ladle, repeat until all the liquid has been used. Season with sea salt to taste.

3. Serve warm.

*See Vegetable Stock recipe NS (page 210).

▶ SERVES 4

2 teaspoons olive oil

½ cup finely diced white onion

1 cup forbidden black rice

Sea salt, to taste

2 cups Vegetable Stock* (or carton organic)

¾ cup almond milk

Herbed Quinoa 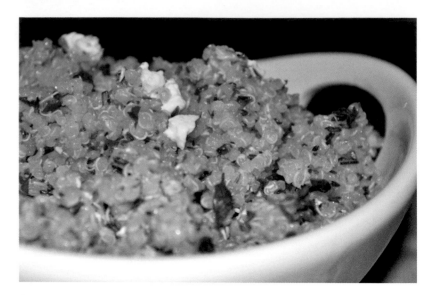 NS

1 cup quinoa

1 cup Vegetable Stock*

1 cup water

1 tablespoon fresh rosemary

1 tablespoon fresh thyme

1 tablespoon fresh parsley

½ teaspoon lemon zest

2 tablespoons flaxseeds

¼ cup crumbled feta cheese

Sea salt, to taste

1. Combine quinoa, stock, and water in a pot. Bring to a boil, reduce heat, and simmer for 10 to 12 minutes.

2. Fluff cooked quinoa with a fork, and toss with rosemary, thyme, parsley, lemon zest, flaxseeds, and feta cheese.

3. Season with salt and serve warm.

*See Vegetable Stock recipe NS (page 210).

▶ SERVES 4

EAT RIGHT FOR YOUR TYPE PERSONALIZED COOKBOOK

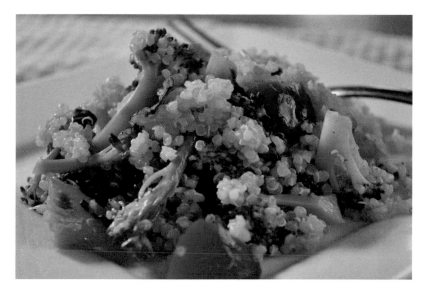

Crisp-Tender Veggie Quinoa

1 small head broccoli

1 bunch broccolini

2 (4-inch) pieces lemongrass

1 cup quinoa

2 cups water

2 teaspoons olive oil

1 cup corn (NS substitute diced red bell pepper)

2 teaspoon lemon zest

Sea salt, to taste

1 tablespoon lemon zest

1. Chop broccoli and broccolini into bite-size pieces. Bring a large pot of water to a boil, and drop broccoli and broccolini in to cook for 3 minutes. Remove with a slotted spoon, and place in an ice bath (a large bowl of water and ice) to stop the cooking process. Drain and set aside on a kitchen towel.

2. Remove white bottom off the lemongrass and hit the stalk with the back of a knife to bruise and bring out its flavors.

3. Bring quinoa and water to a boil with a pinch of salt, reduce heat to simmer, and add lemongrass. Let cook 12 minutes until quinoa has absorbed all of the liquid and has become tender. Fluff quinoa with a fork, remove, and discard lemongrass.

4. Heat olive oil in a large skillet over medium heat. Sauté corn, broccoli, and broccolini for 2 to 3 minutes. Toss vegetables with cooked quinoa, lemon zest, and sea salt, to taste.

5. Serve warm or cold.

▶ SERVES 6

 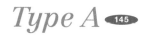

Mint and Pumpkin Tabbouleh

NS

1½ cups finely diced pumpkin

3 tablespoons plus 2 teaspoons olive oil, divided

Sea salt, to taste

1 cup quinoa, raw

2 cups water

4 cups torn kale

1 tablespoon lemon juice

1 tablespoon lemon zest

2 cloves garlic, minced

¾ cup mint

2 cups parsley

1. Preheat oven to 400 degrees.

2. Carefully peel and dice pumpkin into small cubes, and toss with 2 teaspoons olive oil and a dash of sea salt. Place in a single layer on a baking sheet and bake 40 to 45 minutes, until pumpkin is tender and slightly browned on the bottoms and edges. Set aside to cool.

3. Cook quinoa in water and with dash of sea salt. Bring to a boil. Reduce heat, and simmer for 10 minutes. Leave the cover on, and let sit an additional 4 to 5 minutes. Fluff with a fork, and set aside to cool.

4. Place kale on a baking sheet, drizzle with 2 teaspoons olive oil and sprinkle with sea salt. Bake for 10 to 12 minutes until kale pieces are crispy.

5. Whisk remaining olive oil, lemon juice, zest, and garlic in the bottom of a large bowl. Toss with mint, parsley, pumpkin, cooked quinoa, and kale until dressing is evenly distributed.

6. Serve room temperature or chilled.

▶ SERVES 6

Roasted Escarole NS

2 heads escarole,
washed and dried

2 teaspoons olive oil

¼ teaspoon large-grain
sea salt

1. Preheat oven to 375 degrees.

2. Trim woody stems off the bottom of escarole and discard, and give the leaves a rough chop. Toss with olive oil and season with sea salt.

3. Spread escarole evenly across two baking sheets and bake for 10 to 12 minutes. Turn after 5 minutes, to help the escarole become crispy. Escarole should be dark green, wilted, and have crispy, slightly browned edges.

4. Serve immediately.

▶ SERVES 4

 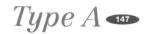

Creamy Rice Polenta (NS)

½ cup brown rice farina
1 teaspoon dried parsley
¼ cup mozzarella cheese
2 teaspoons olive oil
½ teaspoon onion powder

1. Cook brown rice farina according to package instructions. Two minutes before farina is finished cooking, add remaining ingredients, stirring constantly.

2. Serve immediately.

▶ SERVES 2

tip: If polenta is ready before the rest of your meal and becomes too thick, simply add warm water 1 tablespoon at a time until desired consistency is achieved.

EAT RIGHT FOR YOUR TYPE PERSONALIZED COOKBOOK

Snacks

Cheese Toast NS ■ *Summer Squash Salsa* NS ■ *Crudités and Creamy Goat Cheese Dip* NS ■ *Adzuki Hummus* NS ■ *Flax Crackers* NS ■ *Curried Egg Salad* NS ■ *Farmer Cheese and Beet-Endive Cups* NS ■ *Marinated Mozzarella* NS ■ *Rosemary-Nut Mix* NS ■ *Broccolini Wrapped with Crispy Walnut Bacon* NS ■ *Artichoke Bruschetta* NS ■ *Crispy Spring Veggie Cakes* NS ■ *Homemade Applesauce* NS ■ *Stone-Fruit Salad with Mint-Lime Dressing* NS ■ *Pear and Apple Chips* NS ■ *Baked Grapefruit with Honey and Cinnamon* NS ■ *Grilled Pineapple with Cinnamon Syrup* NS ■ *Peanut Butter–Rice Cakes with Mini Chips* NS ■ *Carob–Walnut Butter–Stuffed Figs* NS

Snacks tend to be the most difficult place for most people to get creative and come up with new ideas that are not overly complicated. Hopefully you will come across a few new options that will make snacking easier, tastier, and healthier. There are also a few snacks that translate well as appetizers if you like entertaining or have a little extra time to prepare something special.

Cheese Toast NS

2 slices spelt bread

1 clove garlic, halved

2 teaspoons olive oil

2 thin slices fresh mozzarella cheese

½ teaspoon dried oregano

1. Preheat oven or toaster to broil on high.

2. Lightly toast bread and rub halved garlic cut side down on toast, drizzle with olive oil, top with mozzarella cheese, and garnish with oregano.

3. Place cheese toast under the broiler for 1 to 2 minutes or until cheese is melted and bubbling. Keep an eye on the toast so the cheese does not burn.

4. Serve warm.

▶ SERVES 4

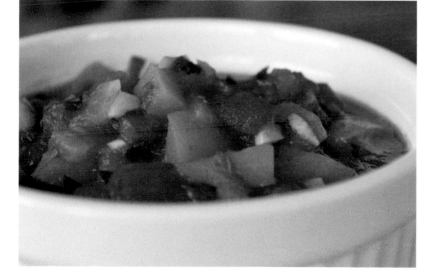
1. Heat olive oil in a 2-quart pot over medium heat. Sauté onion and garlic for 8 to 10 minutes.

2. Add parsnips and zucchini, and sauté until tender, about 10 minutes.

3. Add butternut squash puree, stock, and sage. Bring to a gentle boil, and let simmer 5 minutes.

4. Season with sea salt, and serve as a warm salsa, or let cool in refrigerator and serve chilled.

*See Vegetable Stock NS recipe (page 210).

▶ SERVES 4

1 cup diced sweet onion

1 large garlic clove, minced

2 teaspoons olive oil

1 large parsnip, peeled and diced into ½-inch cubes

2 medium zucchini, diced into ½-inch cubes

1 cup butternut squash puree

½ cup Vegetable Stock*

1 tablespoon chopped fresh sage

Sea salt, to taste

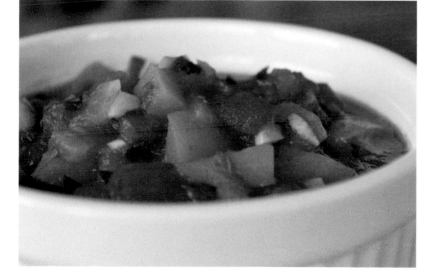

Crudités and Creamy Goat Cheese Dip NS

dip:

4 ounces soft goat cheese

2 tablespoons chopped dill

2 teaspoons agave

½ teaspoon sea salt

1 tablespoon lemon juice

1 tablespoon almond milk

crudités:

Baby carrots

Broccoli florets

Kohlrabi sticks

1. Whisk all dip ingredients in a bowl until smooth and seasonings are fully incorporated.

2. Spoon into a serving dish and plate with crudités.

▶ SERVES 4

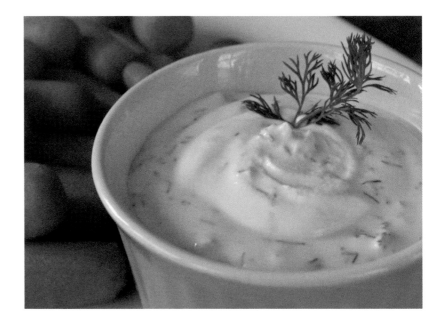

EAT RIGHT FOR YOUR TYPE PERSONALIZED COOKBOOK

1. Put all ingredients in a food processor or a mini chopper, and puree until smooth and creamy. Serve with Flax Crackers NS (page 155) or crudités.

▶ **SERVES 4**

1½ cups cooked (or canned) adzuki beans, drained and rinsed

½ cup chopped fresh basil

2 tablespoons chopped fresh parsley

1 clove garlic, minced

2 teaspoons olive oil

1 tablespoon walnuts

1 teaspoon lemon zest

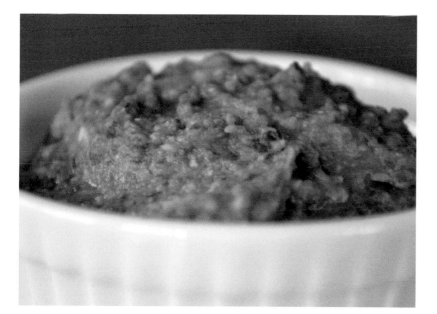

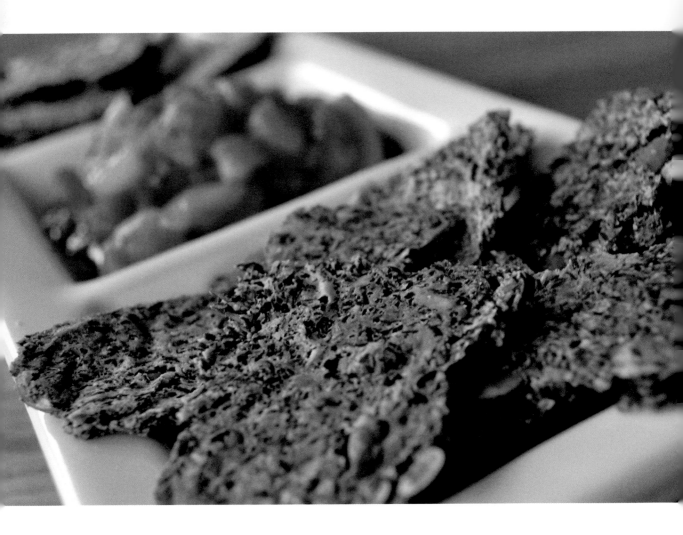

1. Combine flaxseeds with water, stir, and set aside for 15 minutes. Flax will become thick and goopy.

2. Preheat oven to 200 degrees. Line a baking sheet with parchment paper and set aside.

3. Add remaining ingredients to soaked flaxseeds, stirring to combine. Mixture will be slightly thicker in consistency than cake batter. Pour flax mixture onto the center of prepared baking sheet. Spray an offset spatula with cooking spray or coat with olive oil to help you spread the flax mixture without sticking. Spread the mixture in a thin layer as evenly as possible across the whole baking sheet.

4. Bake for 2 hours. Crackers will solidify at this point and be slightly rubbery in texture.

5. Increase the oven temperature to 400, and bake 10 minutes to make the crackers crispy. Carefully flip the crackers, and bake an additional 5 to 6 minutes on the opposite side. When done, crackers will be hardened and crispy on both sides. Let cool, and break apart into pieces the size of tortilla chips.

6. Serve at room temperature, and store in a cool, dry place or in the freezer.

▶ SERVES 4

1 cup coarsely ground flaxseeds

⅔ cup hot water

¼ teaspoon sea salt

¼ cup pepitas (pumpkin seeds)

3 tablespoons almond flour

tip: Whole flaxseeds will last longer than ground, so buy whole and grind in a coffee grinder or food processor when needed to maximize shelf life.

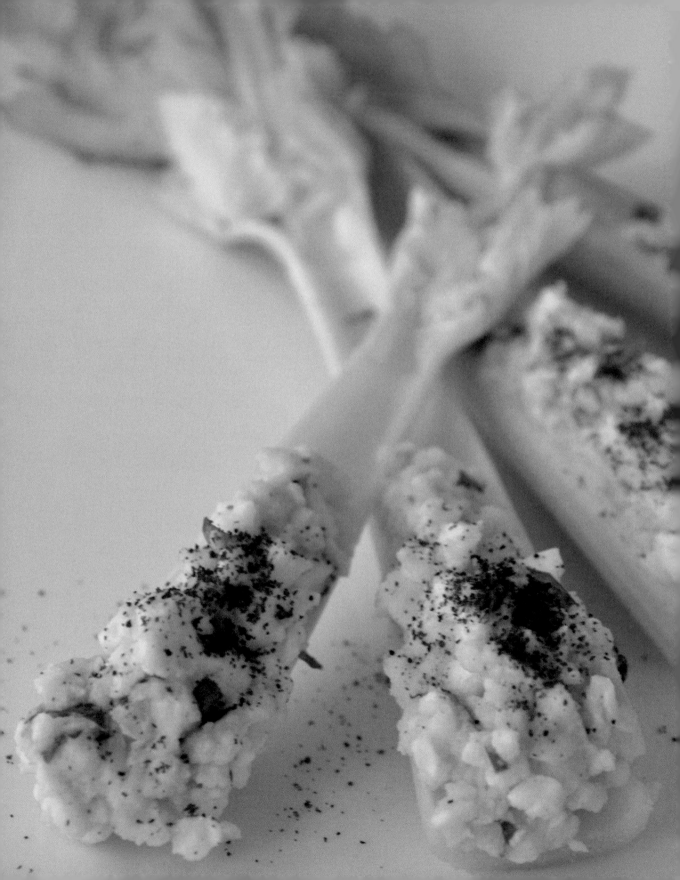

Curried Egg Salad NS

1. Place eggs in a saucepan and cover with cold water. Bring to a boil and turn off the heat. Set a timer for 14 minutes and when done, rinse eggs under cold water. Peel eggs, chop, and place them in a large bowl.

2. Add remaining ingredients to the bowl with the eggs and toss to combine.

3. Serve on celery sticks or between slices of brown rice toast.

▶ SERVES 4

4 large eggs

½ teaspoon dried mustard

1 tablespoon fresh chopped parsley

¼ teaspoon sea salt

½ teaspoon curry powder

⅛ teaspoon turmeric

2 teaspoons olive oil

2 teaspoons lemon juice

Farmer Cheese and Beet-Endive Cups NS

2 medium orange beets
2 medium red beets
2 teaspoons olive oil
¼ cup farmer cheese
¼ cup chopped walnuts
1 teaspoon lemon juice
Sea salt, to taste
2 heads endive

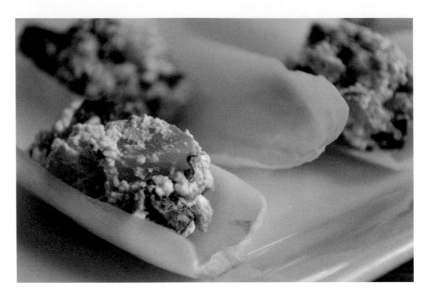

1. Preheat oven to 400 degrees. Line a baking sheet with tinfoil and set aside.

2. Trim tops and bottoms off beets and scrub clean. Place beets on prepared baking sheet, drizzle with olive oil and bake for 60 to 65 minutes, or until easily pierced with a knife.

3. Let beets cool for 10 minutes then carefully remove skin with a paring knife, and dice in ½-inch cubes. Place in bowl with farmer cheese, walnuts, and lemon juice and mix gently to combine. Season, to taste, with sea salt.

4. Spoon about 2 teaspoons of filling onto each endive leaf.

5. Serve immediately, or chill, covered, in the refrigerator until ready to serve.

▶ SERVES 4

tip: Store-bought, precooked beets, either canned or in vacuum-sealed packages in the produce department can be substituted in this recipe, but beets from a can tend to lose a great deal of flavor and sweetness.

EAT RIGHT FOR YOUR TYPE PERSONALIZED COOKBOOK

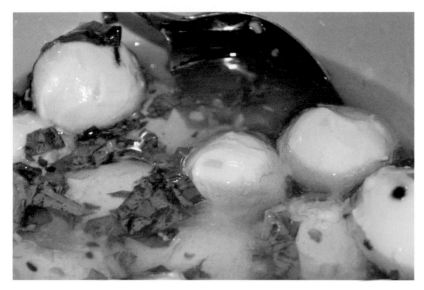

Marinated Mozzarella

NS

½ cup extra virgin olive oil

1 teaspoon large-grain sea salt

2 cloves garlic, minced

2 tablespoons chopped basil

2 kalamata olives, finely diced

1 pound fresh mozzarella balls

1. Place olive oil, sea salt, garlic, basil, and olives in a medium-size bowl, stirring to combine.

Add mozzarella balls, toss to coat, and refrigerate for 2 hours or more. Remove from refrigerator 15 minutes before serving, to allow oil to come to room temperature.

2. Mozzarella balls will keep in the refrigerator for up to 1 week.

▶ SERVES 4

tip: If you cannot find individually portioned, miniature mozzarella balls, buy one large ball of fresh cheese and cut into 1–2-inch pieces as a substitute.

 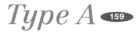

Rosemary-Nut Mix NS

2 tablespoons fresh rosemary

½ teaspoon salt

1 tablespoon maple syrup

2 teaspoons ghee

1 cup black walnuts

½ cup peanuts

½ cup pepitas (pumpkin seeds)

1. Preheat oven to 325 degrees.

2. Toss all ingredients in a bowl and spread on a baking sheet. Bake for 25 minutes, tossing once halfway through. When done, nuts will be aromatic and lightly browned. Let cool and spoon into a bowl to serve.

3. Store, covered, in a cool, dry place for up to 1 week.

▶ SERVES 6

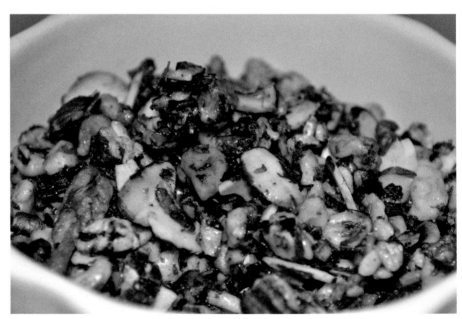

Broccolini Wrapped with Crispy Walnut Bacon NS

1. Preheat oven to 375 degrees.

2. In a small bowl, combine maple syrup, ground ginger, and walnuts. Set aside.

3. Prepare broccolini by cutting off woody ends and separating into individual spears. Toss with olive oil.

4. Slice bacon lengthwise and then into thirds. Wrap 1 piece of bacon around each spear of broccolini and place on a wire rack. Repeat until all broccolini is wrapped.

5. Place wire rack on a baking sheet. Spoon the maple-walnut mixture over the bacon-wrapped broccolini.

6. Bake for 10 to 12 minutes on middle rack. Walnuts will begin to smell nutty and edges of bacon will be crispy.

7. Serve warm.

▶ SERVES 6

2 tablespoons maple syrup

1 teaspoon ground ginger

½ cup finely chopped walnuts

2 bunches broccolini

2 teaspoons olive oil

5 slices nitrate-free/preservative-free turkey bacon

 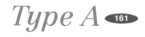

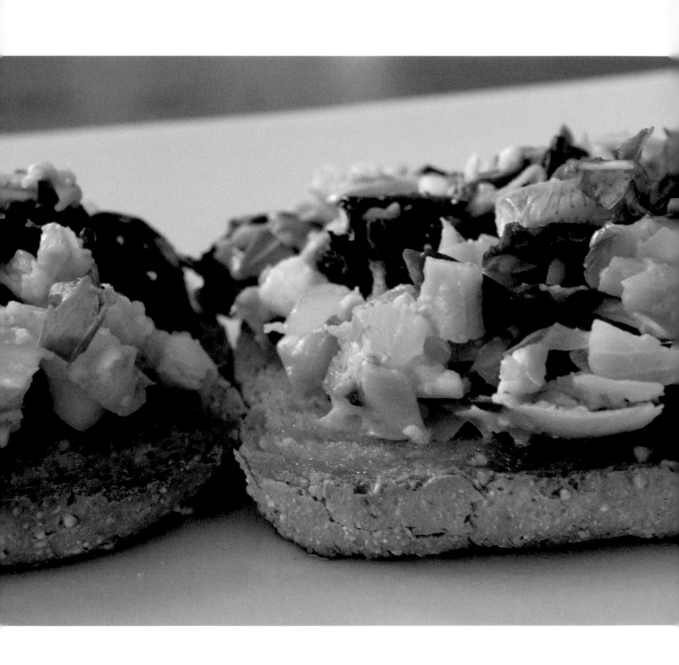

Artichoke Bruschetta

NS

1. Heat a medium skillet over medium heat, and add 2 teaspoons olive oil. Sauté artichokes and onion for 4 to 5 minutes. Season with sea salt and add spinach; sauté an additional 2 to 3 minutes.

2. While the vegetables cook, lightly toast the bread and rub toast with halved garlic. Drizzle toast evenly with remaining olive oil.

3. Remove vegetables from heat, and mix in feta cheese. Spinach will be wilted, and onions and artichoke will be tender and hot.

4. Spoon evenly over toast, and serve warm or at room temperature.

▶ SERVES 2

1 tablespoon olive oil, divided

1 cup frozen artichoke hearts, thawed and chopped

¼ cup finely diced onion

¼ teaspoon sea salt

2 cups chopped spinach

3 slices sprouted wheat or spelt bread

1 clove garlic, halved

¼ cup feta cheese, crumbled

Crispy Spring Veggie Cakes NS

1 cup grated celeriac (celery root)

1 cup grated fennel

2 tablespoons grated onion

2 cups spinach

½ teaspoon lemon zest

1 tablespoon chopped sage

1 large egg

2 tablespoons brown rice flour

⅓ cup bread crumbs*

2 teaspoons olive oil

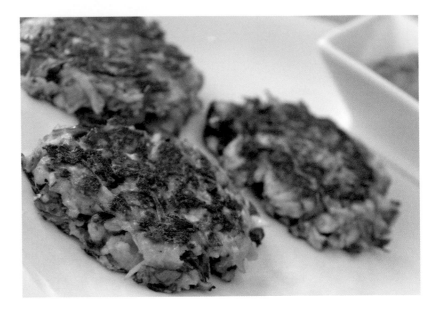

1. Place vegetables in a large bowl. Finely chop spinach, and add to vegetables with lemon zest, sage, egg, flour, and bread crumbs. Toss to combine.

2. In a large skillet over medium heat, heat olive oil. Using an ice cream scoop, spoon vegetable mixture into pan. Allow about 1 inch between each vegetable cake and let cook 2 to 3 minutes. Flip and cook an additional 2 to 3 minutes on the other side. Cakes should be brown and crispy on each side and warm and tender in the center, but cooked through.

3. Serve warm.

*See Basic Bread Crumbs NS recipe (page 210)

▶ SERVES 4

tip: As an alternative serving option, cool and refrigerate to eat as a snack, or for breakfast topped with a poached or fried egg.

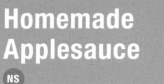
2 organic Red Delicious apples

2 organic Granny Smith apples

1 cinnamon stick

½ cup apple juice

½ cup frozen or fresh organic cranberries

1–2 tablespoons agave

1. Peel apples and dice into 1-inch cubes.

2. Add apples, cinnamon stick, apple juice, and cranberries in a saucepan and bring to a simmer. Add 1 tablespoon agave. Depending on the tartness of the apples and cranberries, an additional tablespoon may be needed. Cook for 30 minutes over medium-low heat or until apples no longer hold their shape.

3. Stir occasionally, remove from heat, and serve warm or chilled.

▶ SERVES 6

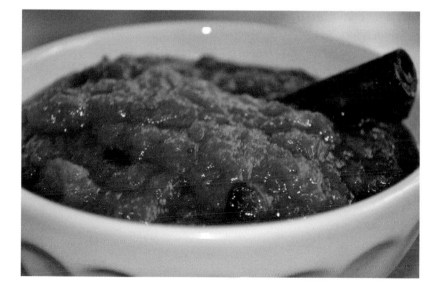

 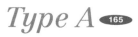

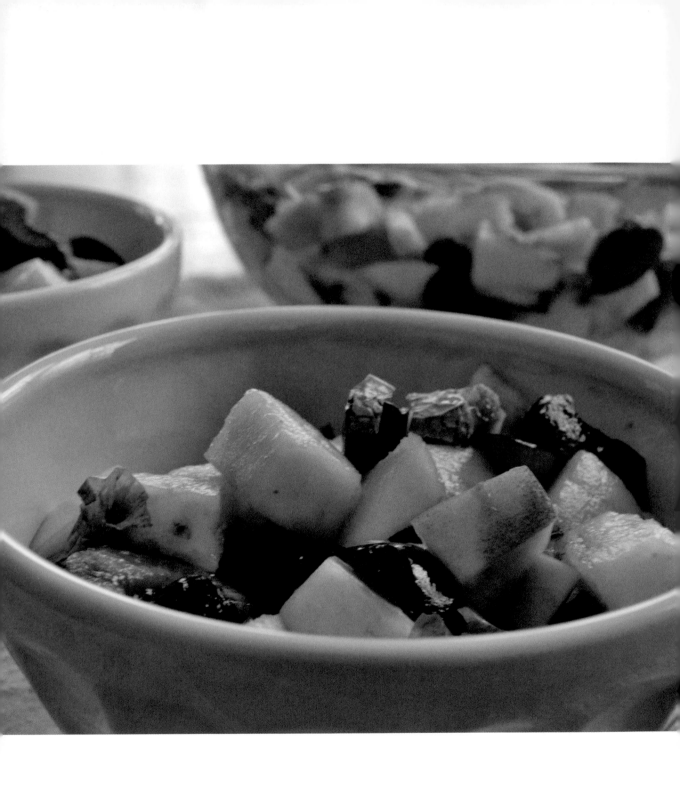

Stone-Fruit Salad with Mint-Lime Dressing NS

½ cup dried cranberries

2 cups fresh cherries, quartered

2 organic peaches

1 pineapple

5 organic apricots

½ cup dried cranberries

Juice and zest of 2 limes

1 teaspoon agave

½ cup finely chopped mint leaves

1. Place dried cranberries in a small bowl. Cover with hot water and steep for 10 minutes, to rehydrate.

2. Dice peaches, pineapple, and apricot into ½-inch pieces. Combine in a large serving bowl, and set aside.

3. Strain cranberries from water, and gently pat dry on a kitchen towel.

4. Whisk lime zest, juice, agave, and mint leaves, and pour over fruit salad. Add cranberries, toss, and serve chilled.

▶ SERVES 6

Pear and Apple Chips

NS

2 Bosc pears
2 Bartlett pears
2 Braeburn apples
¼ teaspoon cinnamon

1. Preheat oven to 225 degrees. Line two baking sheets with parchment paper and set aside.

2. Slice pears and apples in rounds as thinly as you can, or use a mandolin. Place sliced fruit in a single layer on prepared baking sheets and sprinkle evenly with cinnamon.

3. Bake for 2 hours, flipping fruit halfway through cooking.

4. Let cool completely and serve.

▶ SERVES 4

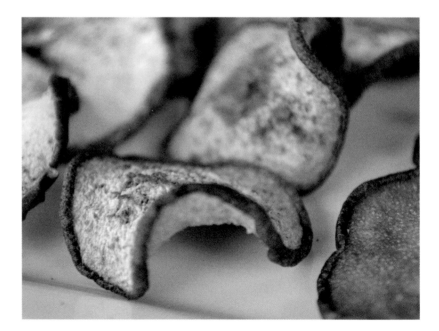

EAT RIGHT FOR YOUR TYPE PERSONALIZED COOKBOOK

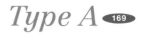
1. Preheat oven to 400 degrees.

2. Trim the rounded bottom of each grapefruit half, just to create a stable base. Place on a baking sheet, flesh side up.

3. Drizzle each half evenly with honey and cinnamon.

4. Bake for 5 to 6 minutes and then broil for 1 to 2 additional minutes until the edges of the grapefruit are browned and the fruit is hot and topping is bubbling.

▶ SERVES 4

2 ruby red grapefruits, halved

2 teaspoons honey

½ teaspoon cinnamon

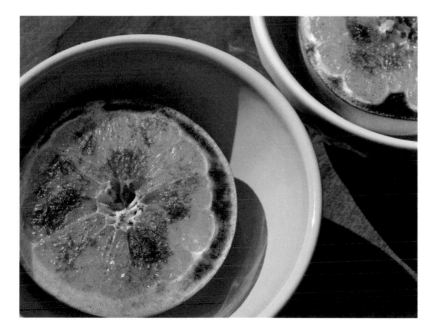

Grilled Pineapple with Cinnamon Syrup NS

2 teaspoons light olive oil
1 fresh pineapple
¼ cup Cinnamon Syrup*

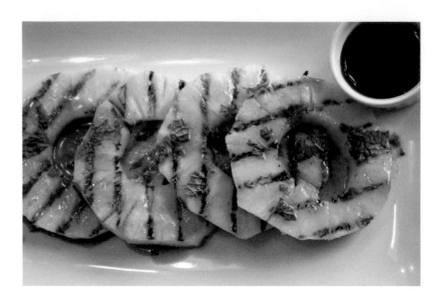

1. Preheat a grill pan over medium heat. Brush grill pan with oil to create a nonstick surface.

2. Remove outer layer of pineapple, core, and slice into rounds.

3. Brush one side of pineapple rounds with Cinnamon Syrup and place syrup-side down on the grill pan. Let cook 2 to 3 minutes, and brush the opposite side with Cinnamon Syrup.

4. Flip and grill an additional 2 to 3 minutes.

5. Serve warm.

*See Cinnamon Syrup NS recipe (page 208).

▶ SERVES 4

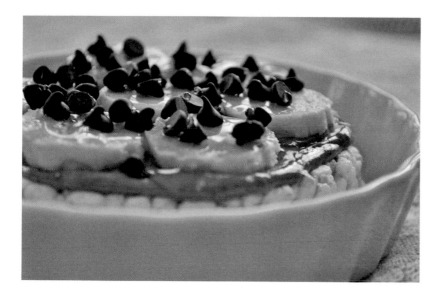

Peanut Butter–Rice Cakes with Mini Chips NS

4 tablespoons peanut butter

2 rice cakes

1 banana, sliced

2 tablespoons mini dark chocolate chips

1 teaspoon honey

1. Smear 2 tablespoons peanut butter on each rice cake and top each with slices from ½ banana, 1 tablespoon chocolate chips, and a drizzle of honey (about ½ teaspoon each).

▶ SERVES 2

Carob–Walnut Butter–Stuffed Figs 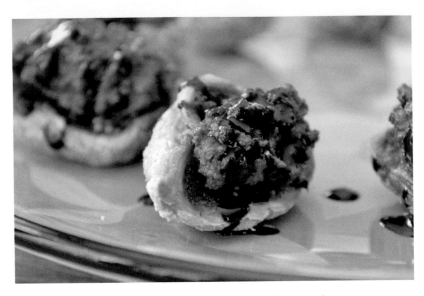 NS

5 fresh or dried figs

¼ cup walnut halves

2 tablespoons pecans

1 tablespoon Carob Extract™ plus more for garnishing*

1 teaspoon olive oil

3 tablespoons hot water

Sea salt, to taste

1. Slice figs in half from stem to base, and set aside.

2. In a food processor, combine walnuts, pecans, Carob Extract, and olive oil. As the processor is running, drizzle in hot water so that the mixture forms a thick paste similar in consistency to natural peanut butter. Season with salt, to taste.

3. Spoon about 1 teaspoon of the nut-butter mixture over each fig half, and drizzle with extra Carob Extract, if desired.

▶ SERVES 2

*Information about purchasing Carob Extract™ can be found in Appendix II: Products (page 233).

Drinks and Beverages

Anytime you start a new diet plan, it is nice to have as many taste and flavor options available to you, especially when you are just getting started. This will help to add diversity to your day in a simple and tasty way. There are plenty of us who have a routine of drinking black tea or soda, and these beverage suggestions can help to substitute for the old habits you are trying to kick. Added also are smoothies, which can spice up your snack or breakfast routine or maybe even replace that milkshake that becomes tempting in the hot, summer months!

Pineapple Spa Water (NS)

2 sprigs mint

6 cups water

4 pineapple slices cut
into ¼-inch rounds

1. Wash mint and place in a large pitcher with water and pineapple slices. Let chill in refrigerator for 2 to 3 hours.

2. Serve chilled.

▶ SERVES 4

Green Detox Juice

1 bunch kale

5 large carrots

3 apples

2-inch piece ginger

1. Run all ingredients through a juicer, one at a time. Pour juice into a tall glass, stirring to combine. Drink immediately for optimal results.

▶ SERVES 4

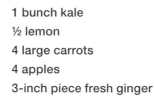
1. Wash and dry vegetables. Cut off tough ends of the kale and carrots, and run kale, lemon, carrots, apples, and ginger through juicer one at a time. Stir together and enjoy.

▶ SERVES 4

1 bunch kale
½ lemon
4 large carrots
4 apples
3-inch piece fresh ginger

tip: Vegetable juices will store in the refrigerator for up to 3 days, but will provide the best nutritional value when consumed immediately after juicing.

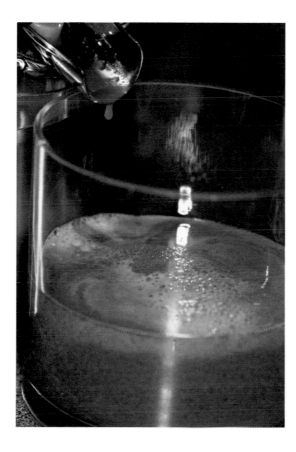

Cooling Chamomile Iced Tea NS

4 cups water
½ cup sliced peaches
1 cup mint leaves
4 chamomile tea bags
¼ cup peach nectar

1. Bring water to a gentle boil and remove from heat.

2. Add peaches, mint leaves, and tea bags, and steep tea for 4 to 5 minutes. Remove tea bags and let cool, then refrigerate until chilled, about 1 hour.

3. Add peach nectar, stir, and serve over ice.

▶ SERVES 4

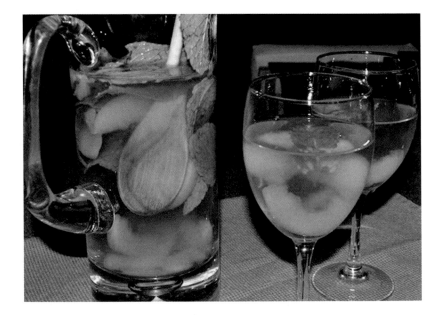

EAT RIGHT FOR YOUR TYPE PERSONALIZED COOKBOOK

Matcha Mojito Tea (NS)

1. Heat water until it is almost at a boil. Add mint and lime juice and zest. Let steep, covered for 5 minutes.

2. Spoon matcha powder into a heat-safe, glass pitcher, and gradually pour water mixture over the matcha, whisking continuously. Strain the mint and zest out of the tea.

3. Add honey and serve.

▶ SERVES 4

6 cups water
1 cup fresh mint
Juice and zest of 1 lime
2 teaspoons matcha powder
1 tablespoon honey

featured ingredient

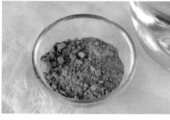

matcha

Matcha is a powdered form of green tea. Once tea leaves are sun dried, they are finely ground and then whisked into not-yet boiling water. Matcha was originally used as a ceremonial tea in Japan, and has just recently become a popular trend in the United States. Because drinking matcha means ingesting all of the tea leaf instead of what is steeped from the leaves, you are consuming a greatly increased amount of antioxidants. Matcha can also be used in baked goods such as cookies and cakes.

 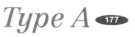

Sweet Basil and Ginger Tea (NS)

4 cups water

2-inch piece fresh ginger, roughly chopped

¼ cup torn basil leaves

1 teaspoon agave nectar

1. Bring water to a boil with ginger, remove from heat, and add basil leaves. Let steep at least 3 minutes. Stir in agave and serve warm.

▶ SERVES 2

Chai Soy Iced Coffee (NS)

5 cups prepared coffee

1 whole clove

1 cinnamon stick

¼ teaspoon dried ginger

⅛ teaspoon ground cardamom

2 tablespoons agave

½ cup soy milk

1. Pour prepared coffee into a saucepan with clove, cinnamon stick, ginger, cardamom, and agave.

2. Warm ingredients over medium-low heat for 8 to 10 minutes, stirring occasionally.

3. Remove cinnamon stick and clove, and remove mixture from heat. Let cool, and then place in the refrigerator until cold, about 1 hour.

4. Once chilled, pour into a large glass pitcher, and add soy milk (add additional soy milk to suit your preference).

5. Serve over ice in chilled glasses.

▶ SERVES 4

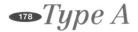 *Type A*

EAT RIGHT FOR YOUR TYPE PERSONALIZED COOKBOOK

1. Combine all ingredients in a blender and blend until smooth. Pour into 2 glasses, and serve cold.

▶ SERVES 2

*Information about purchasing Protein Blend™ Powder—Type A can be found in Appendix II: Products (page 233).

½ cup raspberries

½ cup pineapple

¾ cup blueberries

1 cup torn kale

1 cup soy milk

2 tablespoons peanut butter

2 teaspoons agave

1 tablespoon flaxseeds

2 scoops Protein Blend™ Powder—Type A*

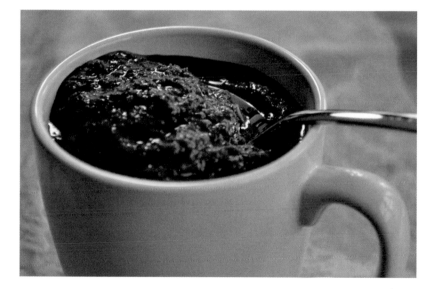

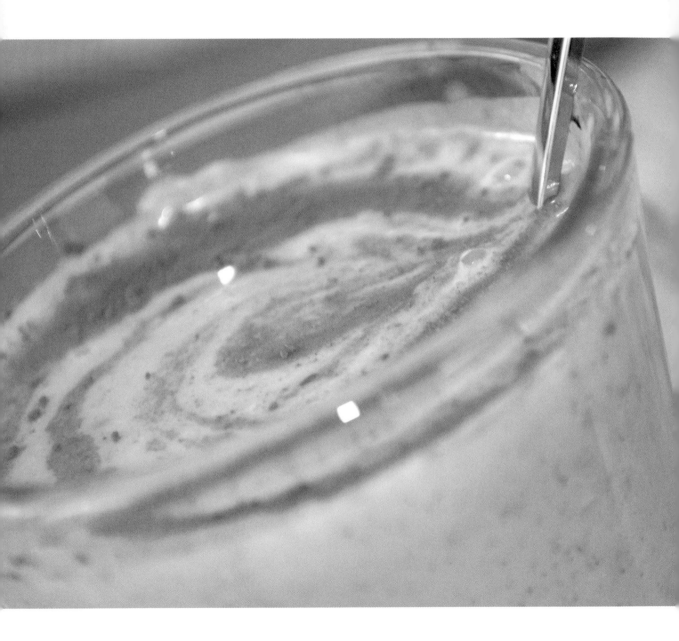

Creamy Peanut Butter Smoothie (NS)

1. Combine all ingredients in a food processor and blend, or use an immersion blender. For easier blending, add liquid to the food processor first. Serve chilled.

▶ SERVES 2

*Information about purchasing Protein Blend™ Powder—Type A can be found in Appendix II: Products (page 233).

4 prunes

2 tablespoons Protein Blend™ Powder—Type A*

8 ounces soy milk

¼ cup avocado, mashed

1 tablespoon flaxseeds

1½ tablespoons peanut butter

Tropical Kale Smoothie NS

1 cup diced frozen pineapple

⅓ cup sliced frozen peaches

¼ cup frozen kale

¾ cup grapefruit juice

2 teaspoons agave

2 tablespoons Protein Blend™ Powder—Type A*

½ teaspoon ground cinnamon

1. Place all ingredients in a blender and blend until smooth. If you have an immersion blender, place all ingredients in a large blender cup and blend until smooth.

▶ SERVES 4

*Information about purchasing Protein Blend™ Powder—Type A can be found in Appendix II: Products (page 233).

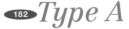

Desserts

What is a cookbook without desserts? The best way to stick to any kind of diet, even ones not meant for weight loss, is to have realistic options for indulging your sweet tooth once in a while. Although these recipes sound indulgent, they are written to be as healthful as possible while still feeling like a satisfying dessert. Whenever possible, use agave or molasses as a sweetener, include allowable grains, limit fats, and feel free to use chocolate.

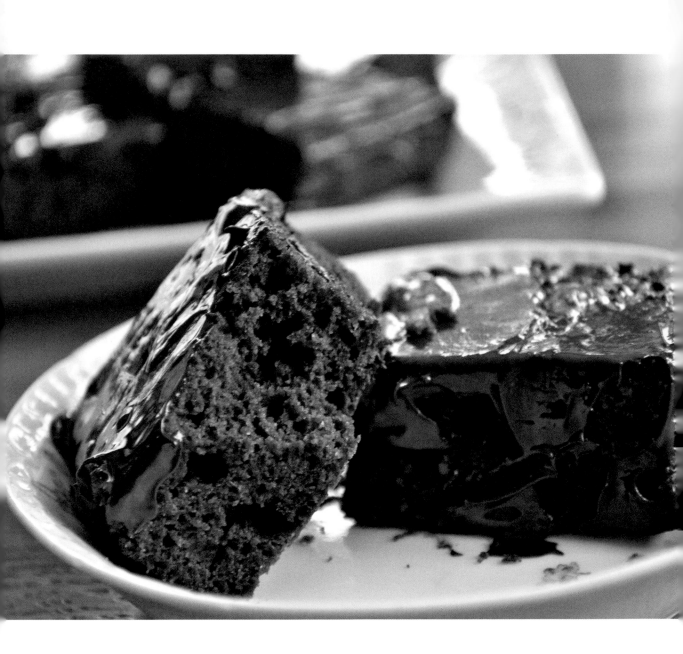

Deep-Chocolate Brownies NS

1. Preheat oven to 350 degrees. Grease an 8"x 8" baking dish and set aside.

2. In a large bowl, combine dry ingredients. Set aside.

3. In a separate bowl, whisk eggs, applesauce, ghee, and agave. Add the egg mixture to the dry mixture and stir to combine.

4. Melt chocolate over a double boiler. If you do not have a double boiler, set a glass bowl on top of a small saucepan filled one-third of the way with water (water should not be touching the bowl). Bring the water to a boil and add shaved chocolate. Let melt and remove from heat. Add chocolate and ¼ cup warm water to batter, stirring to combine.

5. Pour batter into prepared pan and bake for 30 to 35 minutes or until firm to the touch and a cake tester comes out clean.

6. Remove from oven, and turn off the heat. Pour chocolate chips over the top of the brownies, and place back into the oven for 2 to 3 minutes. Use an offset spatula to spread melted chips evenly across the top of the brownies.

7. Let cool for 10 minutes, slice, and serve warm. Brownies will keep in a cool, dry place up to 2 days or in the freezer for up to 1 month.

▶ SERVES 8

1 cup spelt flour
½ cup oat flour
1 teaspoon baking powder
½ teaspoon sea salt
2 tablespoons cocoa powder
2 eggs
¼ cup applesauce
3 tablespoons ghee, melted and cooled, or light olive oil
½ cup agave
2 ounces 100 percent dark chocolate, shaved
¼ cup warm water
½ cup chocolate chips

Cherry-Chocolate Fondue (NS)

2 ounces 100 percent
dark chocolate

2 tablespoons agave

1 cup cherry juice

1 tablespoon cherry jam

2 teaspoons ghee

fruit for dipping:

1 cup diced pineapple

1 cup dried apricot

1 cup sliced apples

1. Shave chocolate into a mixing bowl.

2. In a saucepan, bring agave, juice, jam, and ghee to a low boil and remove from heat. Pour mixture over chocolate and stir to combine.

3. Serve with fruit for dipping.

▶ SERVES 6

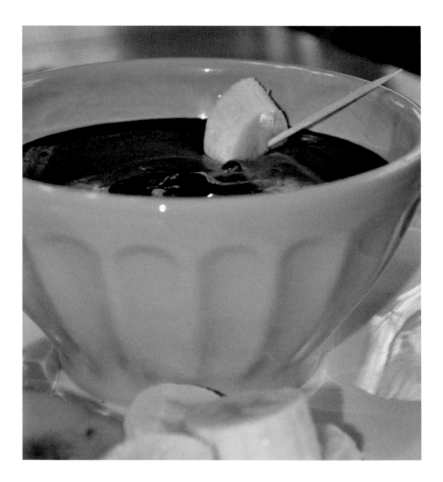

EAT RIGHT FOR YOUR TYPE PERSONALIZED COOKBOOK

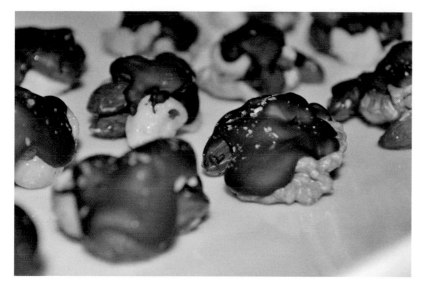

Chocolate Salted Nut Clusters NS

1 cup whole almonds

½ cup quartered walnuts

½ cup halved macadamia nuts

2 teaspoons blackstrap molasses

1 teaspoon agave

½ cup chocolate chips

1 teaspoon large grain sea salt

1. Preheat oven to 350 degrees.

2. Place almonds, walnuts, and macadamia nuts in a medium bowl, and toss to combine. Set aside.

3. In a small saucepan, heat molasses and agave for 30 seconds, just until melted. Drizzle over nuts and toss.

4. Very gently, drop nut clusters by tablespoonful into mini cupcake pans coated with nonstick spray. Place cupcake pan in the oven for 8 to 10 minutes.

5. Remove and let cool. Once cool, place in the freezer for at least 10 minutes.

6. Melt chocolate over a double boiler. Note that water in the double boiler should never touch the base of the top pan to prevent burning.

7. Remove nut clusters from the freezer and spoon melted chocolate over the top, sprinkle evenly with sea salt, and freeze for an additional 10 minutes.

8. Serve cold or at room temperature. Keep in an airtight glass container for up to 1 week or freeze for 1 month.

▶ SERVES 6

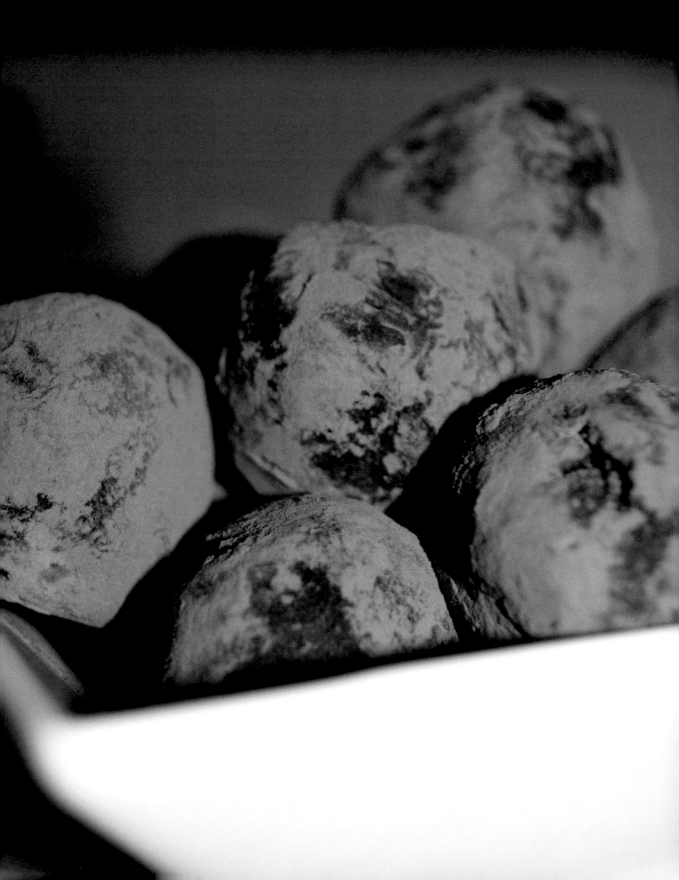

8 ounces 100 percent dark chocolate

¼ cup ghee

⅔ cup agave

½ cup almond or soy milk

⅛ teaspoon large-grain sea salt

3 tablespoons cocoa powder

1. Shave chocolate and place in a medium bowl. Warm ghee, agave, milk, and salt in a saucepan. Once warm, pour mixture over chocolate, whisking continuously until smooth.

2. Cool mixture to room temperature, then cover tightly and refrigerate until chocolate is firm, about 2 to 3 hours.

3. Using a tablespoon or melon baller, scoop out truffles and roll into balls (slightly smaller than a golf ball), then gently roll around in cocoa powder. Refrigerate until ready to serve.

4. Store in an airtight container in the refrigerator for up to 1 week.

▶ SERVES 6

featured ingredient

agave nectar

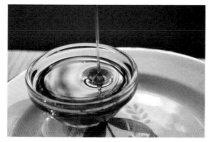

Agave is a natural sweetener derived from the agave plant, commonly found in the southwestern areas of America and in Mexico. Agave is most known for its role as the base ingredient of tequila. It can be used in baking and cooking in place of sugar, however the agave to sugar ratio is not 1:1 because it is a liquid. Agave has a mild taste akin to that of honey, but much less noticeable.

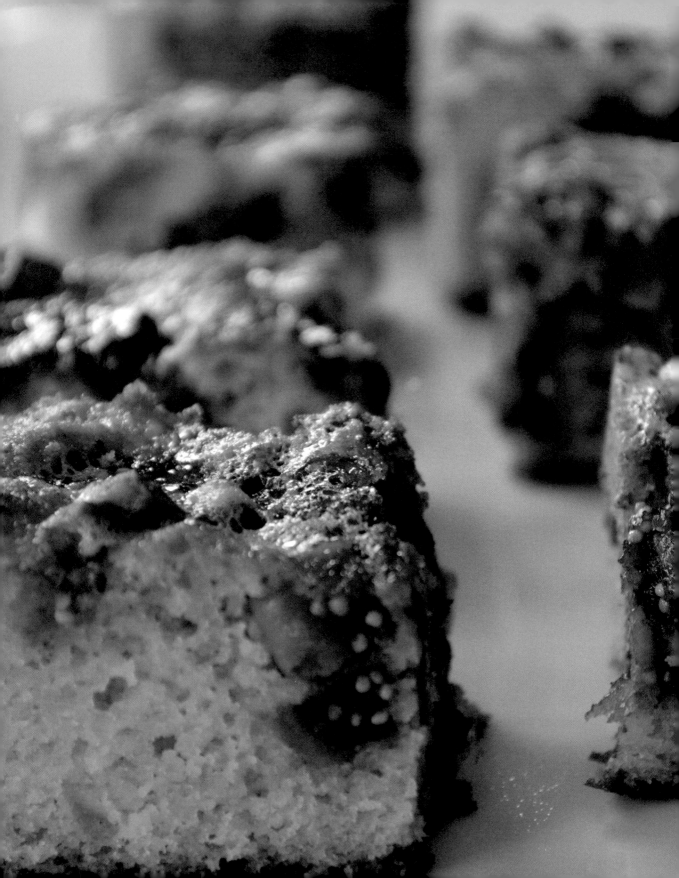

Fig Bars NS

1. Preheat oven to 350 degrees. Grease a 9" x 11" baking dish and set aside.

2. Combine flours with baking powder and sea salt in a large bowl. Mix just until combined.

3. Whisk whole eggs with cooled ghee, and add to flour mixture, mixing until smooth and free of lumps.

4. In a clean, dry glass bowl, beat egg whites until they form stiff peaks. Fold egg whites into batter, one-third at a time.

5. Pour batter into baking dish, and bake for about 15 minutes, until crust begins to firm.

6. While the crust cooks, combine all topping ingredients in a large bowl, mixing until well combined.

7. Remove par-baked crust from oven. Spoon topping mixture over crust and spread evenly. Return to the oven, and bake an additional 35 to 40 minutes, or until a cake tester comes out clean.

8. Serve warm or at room temperature. Bars will keep in a cool, dry place for 1 to 2 days, or freeze for up to 1 month.

▶ SERVES 12

⅔ cup brown rice flour

¼ cup millet flour

¼ cup arrowroot flour

1 teaspoon baking powder

½ teaspoon sea salt

2 large eggs

4 tablespoons ghee, melted and cooled, plus more for greasing

2 large egg whites

topping:

½ cup fig jam

½ cup dried figs, cut into ½-inch dice

¼ cup agave

2 eggs, slightly beaten

1 egg white

2 teaspoons lemon zest

½ teaspoon ground cinnamon

⅛ teaspoon ground cloves

2 tablespoons brown rice flour

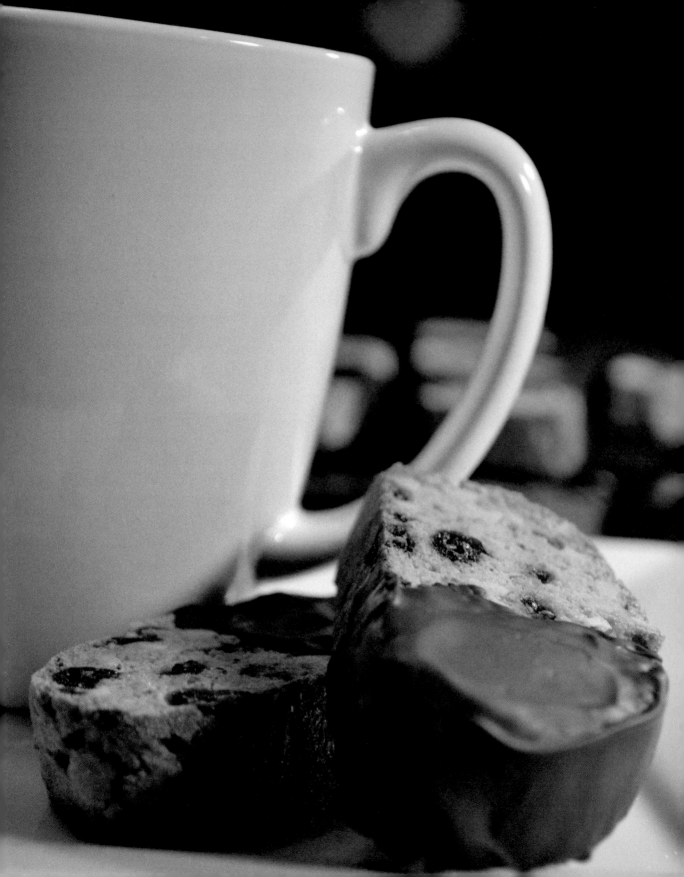

Almond-Cranberry Biscotti NS

1. Preheat oven to 350 degrees. Line an 11" x 17" baking sheet with parchment paper and set aside.

2. In a small bowl, pour hot water over cranberries to rehydrate; let steep for 10 minutes.

3. In a large bowl, mix together flours, baking powder, salt, and almonds. Set aside.

4. In a separate bowl, whisk eggs, lemon zest, agave, and apricot jam. Add egg mixture to dry ingredients, stirring just until combined. Drain cranberries and pat dry. Toss cranberries into biscotti dough.

5. Gather dough into a ball and place on floured work surface. Gently roll dough with hands into a long, flat log, about the length of your baking sheet. Place on prepared baking sheet and bake for 30 minutes. Remove from oven, and let cool 5 minutes. At this point, the biscotti will have the texture of soft bread. Using a serrated knife, cut biscotti on the bias into ¾-inch slices. Place each slice flat on the baking sheet, and bake for an additional 25 minutes, flipping once halfway through baking, so that the cookies will be dry and crunchy all the way through.

6. Remove from oven and let cool on a drying rack. As an optional addition, heat chocolate morsels over a double boiler until melted and silky. Spoon chocolate over half of each cooled biscotti, and let the chocolate cool again.

7. Serve at room temperature. Store in a cool, dry place overnight or in the freezer for up to 1 month.

▶ SERVES 12

¾ cup dried cranberries

1 cup amaranth flour

1½ cups brown rice flour, plus more for rolling

3 teaspoons baking powder

½ teaspoon fine-grain sea salt

1 cup slivered almonds

3 large eggs

1 teaspoon lemon zest

⅓ cup agave

⅓ cup apricot jam

½ cup allergy-free chocolate morsels (optional)

Chocolate Chip Cookies (NS)

½ cup spelt flour

½ cup oat flour

1 teaspoon sea salt

½ teaspoon baking powder

½ teaspoon baking soda

½ cup ghee, softened

½ cup agave

1 tablespoon molasses

1 teaspoon vanilla

½ cup allergy-free chocolate chips

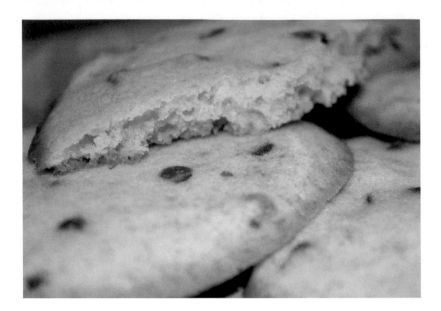

1. Preheat oven to 350 degrees. Line a 15" x 10" baking sheet with parchment paper and set aside.

2. In a large bowl, mix flours with salt, baking powder, and baking soda. Set aside.

3. In a separate bowl, beat softened ghee with agave, molasses, and vanilla until smooth and creamy.

4. Add ghee mixture to flour mixture and stir just until combined and free of lumps. Stir in chocolate chips and, using a tablespoon, spoon cookie dough 2 inches apart, on prepared baking sheet.

5. Bake 12 minutes in the center rack of the oven until dough is cooked and soft with golden edges. Eat warm or let cool on a wire rack. Cookies will keep in a cool, dry place for 1 to 2 days or in the freezer up to 1 month.

▶ SERVES 12

EAT RIGHT FOR YOUR TYPE PERSONALIZED COOKBOOK

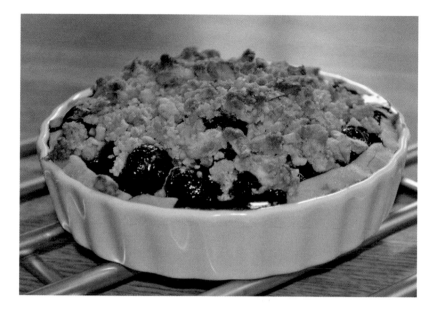

Blueberry Crumble (NS)

crust:

1 cup spelt flour plus more for rolling

¼ teaspoon sea salt

4 tablespoons chilled ghee

4–5 tablespoons ice-cold water

filling:

1 teaspoon lemon zest

¼ teaspoon sea salt

¼ teaspoon cinnamon

⅓ cup agave

¼ teaspoon ginger

2 cups (fresh or frozen) blueberries

topping:

¼ cup finely chopped walnuts

¼ cup spelt flour

2 tablespoons ghee

1 tablespoon agave

1. Preheat oven to 350 degrees.

2. Whisk together spelt flour and salt. Cut cold ghee into small pieces and add to flour mixture. Using a crossing motion with two butter knives or a pastry cutter, incorporate ghee into the flour until the mixture resembles coarse corn meal. Add water, 1 tablespoon at a time, until the dough comes together but is not sticky. Gather dough in your hands and knead until it becomes smooth and pliable. Do not overwork dough; you should still see small pieces of ghee. Cover dough with plastic wrap and refrigerate 1 hour.

3. Roll dough out on a floured surface until about 12 inches in diameter and approximately ⅛-inch thick. Gently press the dough into a 9-inch pie plate, and pinch edges between two fingers to create crimped edges.

4. In a large bowl, stir together filling ingredients just until combined. Spoon into prepared pastry crust.

5. Make topping by combining walnuts and spelt flour in a large bowl. Use your fingers to incorporate the ghee into the dough. Stir in agave and sprinkle on top of blueberry filling.

6. Bake for 25 to 30 minutes.

7. Serve warm.

▶ SERVES 4

Apricot-Cinnamon Charlotte NS

1 teaspoon ghee plus more for greasing

1 teaspoon light olive oil

2 cups diced apricot (fresh or frozen)*

¼ cup dried cranberries

¼ cup dry toasted walnuts

3 large eggs

1 tablespoon soy milk

½ teaspoon cinnamon

8 slices oat, spelt, or soy flour bread

1. Preheat oven to 350 degrees. Grease 2 (12-oz.) ramekins with ghee, and set aside.

2. Heat a large skillet over medium heat, and melt 1 teaspoon of ghee and olive oil. Once hot, add apricots, cranberries, and walnuts. Cook 5 minutes.

3. While the fruit cooks, whisk eggs, soy milk, and cinnamon in a large, flat-bottomed bowl. Set aside.

4. Prepare slice of toast by slicing edges to fit the bottom of your ramekins, and cut so the bread will fit the sides without being too tall or short. Dunk slices of bread in egg mixture, as if making French toast. Line the bottom and edges of prepared ramekins with the egg-soaked bread. Leave two slices of bread for the top.

5. Spoon apricot mixture into the ramekins and top each with 1 slice of toast.

6. Bake for 35 minutes or until golden brown.

▶ SERVES 2

*If apricots are not in season or difficult to find, peaches can be substituted in this recipe.

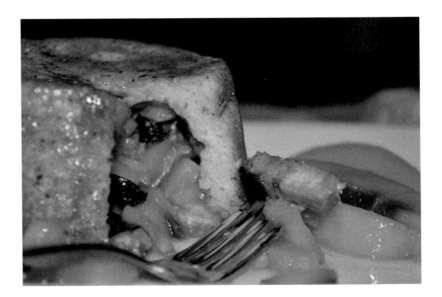

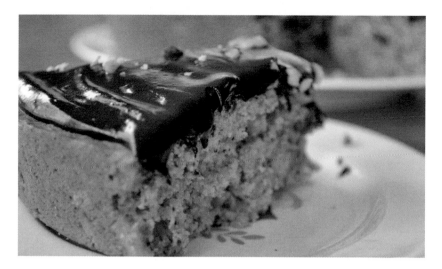

Carrot-Pineapple Cake with Chocolate-Chai Frosting NS

1. Preheat oven to 350 degrees. Grease a 9-inch-round cake pan and set aside.

2. Place shredded carrot and diced pineapple on paper towels to absorb excess liquid.

3. In a large bowl, combine flours, arrowroot starch, baking powder, salt, and cinnamon. Set aside.

4. In a separate bowl, whisk together egg yolks, pineapple, carrots, walnuts, 3 tablespoons ghee, and agave. Add to dry ingredients, stirring to combine.

5. In a dry, glass bowl, beat egg whites until stiff peaks form. Fold egg whites into batter, one-third at a time. Pour into prepared cake pan.

6. Bake 35 to 40 minutes.

7. Prepare chocolate chai frosting: in a small saucepan, heat almond milk, agave, cinnamon, ginger, and allspice for 2 to 3 minutes. Place grated chocolate in a bowl with ghee. Pour almond milk mixture over chocolate and whisk until smooth. Let cool completely. Add cocoa powder, and stir until mixture thickens.

8. Spread frosting on top of the cooled cake and sprinkle with walnuts for garnish. For best results, serve same day or store in a cool, dry place overnight or in the freezer for up to 1 month.

▶ SERVES 8

1 cup shredded carrot

¾ cup diced pineapple

3 tablespoons ghee, melted and cooled, plus more for greasing

1 cup brown rice flour

1 cup millet flour

¼ cup arrowroot starch

3 teaspoons baking powder

1 teaspoon salt

½ teaspoon cinnamon

2 large egg yolks

1 cup finely chopped walnuts

½ cup agave

4 large egg whites

frosting:

½ cup almond milk

4 tablespoons agave

1 teaspoon ground cinnamon

½ teaspoon ground ginger

⅛ teaspoon ground allspice

3 ounces 100 percent dark chocolate, grated

2 tablespoons ghee

2 tablespoons cocoa powder

¼ cup chopped walnuts, for garnish

 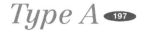

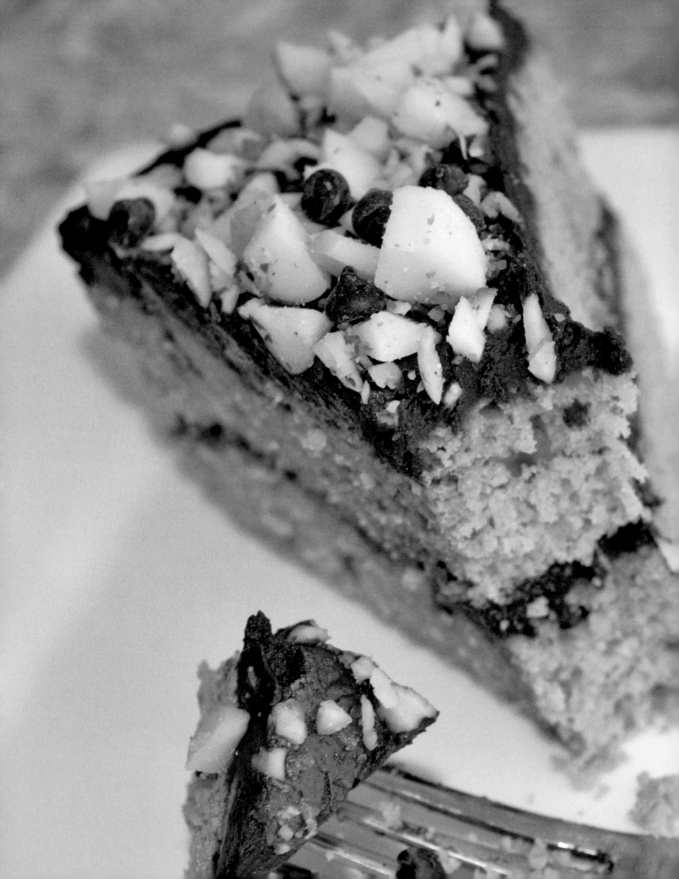

1. Preheat oven to 350 degrees. Grease two 9-inch-round cake pans with butter or ghee, and set aside.

2. In a large bowl, combine matcha, flours, baking powder, salt, and cloves. Set aside.

3. In a separate bowl, whisk together lemon zest, agave, ghee, eggs, egg yolk, and almond milk. Set aside.

4. Place egg whites in a glass, copper, or metal bowl and beat on high until egg whites form stiff peaks, and set aside.

5. Add wet mixture to dry mixture, stirring until well combined and lump-free. Using one-third of the egg white mixture at a time, fold whites gently into the batter.

6. Pour batter evenly into prepared cake pans, and bake in the middle rack of the oven for 25 minutes, until cake is firm and cake tester comes out clean. Let cool in pans for 10 minutes, and remove to wire cooling racks to cool fully.

7. Prepare chocolate frosting by heating almond milk and agave in a small saucepan for 2 to 3 minutes. Place grated chocolate in a bowl with ghee. Pour almond milk mixture over chocolate and stir until smooth. Let cool completely. Add cocoa powder and stir until mixture thickens.

8. Spread slightly less than half the frosting on the first layer of cake, top with the second layer, and use an offset spatula to spread remaining frosting over the top of the second tier of cake. Sprinkle with toasted macadamia nuts and chocolate morsels, and serve.

▶ SERVES 8

1 tablespoon matcha powder

1½ cups brown rice flour

1 cup millet flour

3 teaspoons baking powder

½ teaspoon fine-grain sea salt

¼ teaspoon ground cloves

1 teaspoon lemon zest

½ cup agave

4 tablespoons ghee, melted and cooled, plus 1 tablespoon for greasing

2 large eggs

1 egg yolk

⅓ cup almond milk

3 large egg whites

frosting:

½ cup almond milk

4 tablespoons agave

3 ounces 100 percent dark chocolate, grated

2 tablespoons ghee

2 tablespoons cocoa powder

⅔ cup chopped, toasted macadamia nuts

¼ cup allergy-free chocolate morsels

Buckwheat Crêpes with Raspberry Chutney and Chocolate Syrup

¾ cup buckwheat flour

¼ cup spelt flour

1 tablespoon ghee plus 1 teaspoon, melted (optional)

½ teaspoon fine sea salt

2 large eggs

1½ cups almond or soy milk

raspberry chutney:

1 Bosc pear, diced

1 teaspoon ghee

1 teaspoon lemon zest

½ teaspoon grated fresh ginger

¼ cup sugar-free apricot jam

1 cup halved fresh raspberries, or cranberries can be substituted

¼ cup Chocolate Syrup*

1. Whisk all crêpe ingredients together in a large bowl. Cover and refrigerate for 1 hour.

2. While the batter is chilling, in a medium skillet, heat ghee over medium heat and sauté pear for 3 to 4 minutes, or until slightly browned and tender. Add lemon zest, ginger, and apricot jam, cooking for an additional 30 seconds. Remove from heat and toss with fresh raspberries.

3. Heat a large, low-sided skillet over medium to medium-high heat, and (if not nonstick) brush with remaining melted ghee. Once hot, spoon ¼ cup crêpe batter onto the skillet and quickly turn the skillet to spread batter into a very thin layer. Let cook about 1 minute, or until the edges start to pull away from the skillet and tiny bubbles appear in the center of the crêpe. Using a large, flat spatula or carefully lifting edges with your hands, flip the crêpe and cook an additional minute on the other side.

4. Continue making crêpes until all batter is used. Stack crêpes on a plate and keep warm until serving.

5. Serve warm with chutney and drizzle with chocolate syrup.

▶ SERVES 4

*See Chocolate Syrup recipe (page 207).

EAT RIGHT FOR YOUR TYPE PERSONALIZED COOKBOOK

featured ingredient

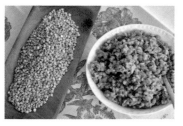

buckwheat

Buckwheat is a gluten-free, pyra-mid-shaped grain that has a slightly sweet, nutty flavor and is high in protein. It is a delicious al-ternative to wheat that pairs per-fectly with fresh fruit and chocolate! Buckwheat can also be eaten as a whole-grain side to any meal, much like rice and quinoa. It is quick to cook and a nutritious varia-tion on your weeknight meal.

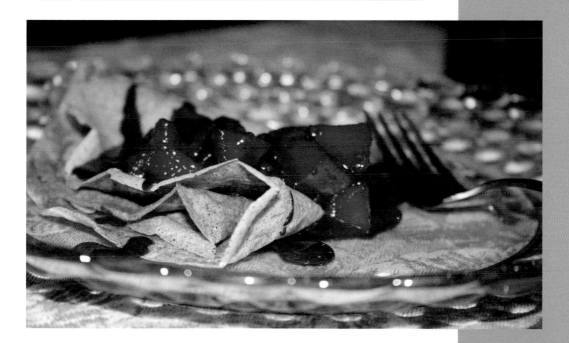

Upside-Down Almond Cake with Apricot Glaze NS

1 cup brown rice flour

½ cup millet flour

½ cup finely ground almond meal

2 teaspoons baking powder

½ teaspoon fine sea salt

½ teaspoon lemon zest

4 large egg whites

2 large egg yolks

½ cup agave

2 tablespoons honey

6 tablespoons ghee, softened

5 tablespoons almond milk

1 cup whole almonds

topping:

2 tablespoons honey

¼ cup sugar-free apricot jam

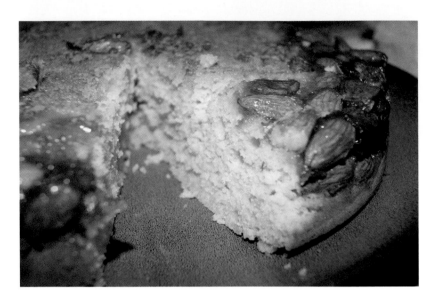

1. Preheat oven to 350 degrees. Grease a round 9-inch cake pan, line with parchment paper, and set aside.

2. In a large bowl, whisk together flours, almond meal, baking powder, and salt. Set aside.

3. In a dry, glass bowl, beat egg whites with a hand mixer until they form stiff peaks, and set aside.

4. In a small bowl, mix egg yolks, agave, honey, ghee, and almond milk, and add to dry mixture. Stir just until combined. Fold egg whites into batter one-third at a time.

5. Scatter almonds evenly on the bottom of the cake pan. In a small saucepan, warm honey and apricot jam for 30 seconds, creating a thin glaze. Slowly pour evenly over almonds in the bottom of the cake pan. Pour batter over almonds and glaze and bake for 40 minutes, or until a cake tester comes out clean.

▶ SERVES 8

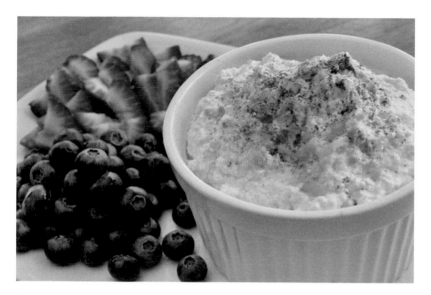

Creamy Berry Ricotta NS

16 ounces organic, part-skim ricotta cheese

¼ teaspoon cinnamon

1 teaspoon lemon zest

2 teaspoons agave

¼ teaspoon sea salt

¾ cup strawberries

¾ cup blueberries

1. In a medium-size bowl, stir together ricotta cheese, cinnamon, lemon zest, agave, and sea salt.

2. Slice strawberries, and use with blueberries to dip, or stir into ricotta mixture.

▶ SERVES 4

 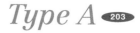

Ginger Rice Pudding (NS)

1 cup brown basmati rice

½ teaspoon sea salt

3½ cups almond milk, divided

1 tablespoon fresh ginger, grated

⅛ teaspoon cardamom (optional)

¼ teaspoon cinnamon

2 large egg yolks

2 tablespoons oat flour

1 tablespoon blackstrap molasses

1 tablespoon maple syrup

½ cup diced, dried apricot (no sugar added)

1. In a medium saucepan, bring 1 cup brown basmati rice, sea salt, and 2 cups almond milk to a boil. Reduce heat to a simmer, cover, and simmer for 50 minutes.

2. In a small saucepan, heat remaining 1½ cups almond milk with ginger, cardamom, if using, and cinnamon until warm. In a small bowl, whisk together egg yolks, flour, molasses, and maple syrup. Temper the egg mixture by adding a ladle of the warm milk to the eggs very slowly and whisking continuously. Once the eggs have been warmed, add the mixture into the warmed milk, and whisk over medium heat until the mixture is thick. The consistency should resemble yogurt when it is ready. Remove from heat, and set aside.

3. When rice is cooked, add apricot and milk mixture to the rice. Let cook an additional 3 to 5 minutes over low heat, stirring continuously. The rice pudding will be thick and creamy.

4. Serve warm.

▶ SERVES 6

Stocks, Condiments, and Sauces

Herb Dressing NS

¼ cup finely chopped
fresh basil

2 tablespoons finely
chopped fresh parsley

2 tablespoons finely
chopped fresh chives

2 small cloves garlic,
minced

½ cup extra virgin olive
oil

⅔ cup fresh-squeezed
lemon juice

Sea salt, to taste

1. Whisk herbs, garlic, olive oil, and lemon juice together in a small bowl, or pour ingredients in a glass jar with a sealable lid and shake vigorously to combine. Season with sea salt, to taste.

2. Store salad dressing in a glass jar or dispenser in the refrigerator for up to 1 week. Recipe can be doubled so you have it ready to go all week.

Citrus Dressing NS

½ cup extra virgin olive
oil

Juice of 2 lemons

Juice of 1 lime

2 tablespoons finely
chopped cilantro

2 teaspoons agave

Sea salt, to taste

1. Whisk olive oil, lemon juice, lime juice, cilantro, and agave together in a small bowl, or pour ingredients in a glass jar with a sealable lid and shake vigorously to combine. Season with sea salt, to taste.

2. Store salad dressing in a glass jar or dispenser in the refrigerator for up to 1 week. Recipe can be doubled so you have it ready to go all week.

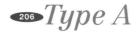

Carrot-Ginger Dressing (NS)

2 medium carrots, chopped

1 tablespoon olive oil

1-inch piece fresh ginger, peeled

1 tablespoon fresh lemon juice

Sea salt, to taste

1. In the food processor, pulse carrots, olive oil, ginger, and lemon juice until a smooth consistency is reached. If the mixture is too thick, add water, 1 tablespoon at a time.

2. Season with sea salt, to taste, and store in a glass container or dispenser in the refrigerator for up to 1 week.

Chocolate Syrup

1 cup agave

2 tablespoons cocoa powder

1. Whisk agave and cocoa powder vigorously in a bowl to incorporate. Once combined, store in a clean, glass dispenser or a glass container to be drizzled over pancakes, fruit, or to add a special treat to smoothies.

2. Store in a cool, dry place for up to 2 weeks.

Tangy Tofu Marinade

1 tablespoon paprika

1 teaspoon mustard powder

¼ teaspoon ground cumin

½ teaspoon large grain sea salt

½ cup olive oil

Juice of 1 lemon

1 tablespoon agave

1. Whisk all ingredients together in small bowl and pour over tofu, vegetables, or poultry for a quick and delicious marinade.

Cinnamon Syrup NS

2 teaspoons butter

1 cup agave

2 teaspoons cinnamon

1. Melt butter in a saucepan over medium-low heat. Add agave and cinnamon, whisking until smooth and combined. Remove from heat and let cool completely.

2. Store in a clean, glass dispenser or container in the refrigerator for up to 2 weeks.

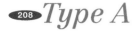

1. Bring all ingredients to a gentle boil in a large stockpot. As the stock boils, use a large spoon to skim foam and impurities off the top and discard. Reduce to a simmer.

2. After 3 hours, remove ingredients from stock and strain into a clean bowl or pot. Let cool (not more than 4 hours), then package and refrigerate.

3. Store in glass containers in the refrigerator for up to 3 days or in the freezer for 2 months.

4. If you want to utilize the cooked meat for salad, casseroles, or to add to your soup, pick the meat off the bones after 1 hour of cooking, cool and refrigerate for another use. Continue to cook the bones and vegetables. The stock will be lighter, but the meat will be viable for other uses (such as in sandwiches, topped on salads, in casseroles, pot pie and so on).

4 pounds chicken or turkey thighs and breast

3 large carrots, peeled and diced

1 celery root, peeled and diced

2 cloves garlic, peeled

1 Vidalia onion, chopped

4 quarts water

2 teaspoons sea salt

3 sprigs fresh thyme

3 sprigs fresh rosemary

5 sprigs parsley

2 bay leaves

Vegetable Stock NS

2 teaspoons olive oil

2 onions, chopped

1 celery root, peeled and chopped

1 cup chopped parsnips

1 cup chopped carrots

3 tomatoes, halved

2 fennel bulbs, chopped

3 bay leaves

1 clove garlic, peeled

5 sprigs parsley

5 sprigs thyme

2 teaspoons sea salt

4 quarts water

1. Heat a large stockpot over medium heat. Add olive oil and sauté onions, celery root, parsnip, carrots, and fennel for 8 to 10 minutes. Add water and remaining ingredients, and bring to a boil.

2. Cover, reduce heat to low, and cook for 30 minutes. Vegetable stock has a quick cooking time, because vegetables give up their flavor quickly, as opposed to meats and bones.

3. Strain stock into a clean pot, and store in the refrigerator for up to 5 days or in the freezer for up to 3 months.

Basic Bread Crumbs NS

4 slices spelt or oat bread

1. Toast slices of bread, and let cool. Pulse cooled toast in a food processor until they become coarse bread crumbs.

2. For flavored bread crumbs, add dried herbs such as parsley, rosemary, thyme, sage, and/or basil.

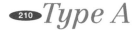

Useful Tools

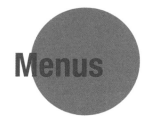

Substitutions

An integral part of acclimating to your new diet is being able to fill the void created by your *Best Avoided* list. Below is a list of substitutions to help you along the way. A number of these substitutions will not directly translate one to another but you will see from recipes in this book how they are adapted to work in place of one another.

BREAD—The beauty about being Type A is that there are many bread options out there for you. The caution here is to read the labels of bread you buy in the store. Many breads claim to be "whole grain oat bread," but contain white flour or some other ingredient that is on your *Avoid* list. I always recommend variety in a healthy diet, so even if you find a great oat bread, try out a spelt, rye, or sprouted wheat bread to mix things up and diversify your nutritional intake.

PASTA—The best pasta you can get is soba, which is a buckwheat-based pasta. Similar to the issue with breads, however, many varieties contain white flour, so make sure you read labels. Whole wheat pasta is also another option, but buckwheat is more *Beneficial* and has a delicious nutty flavor that will pair beautifully with soy-marinated tofu and roasted veggies.

BUTTER—This may be one of those things that is difficult to let go. A terrific alternative is ghee, which is simply clarified butter. When butter is heated, it separates and the lactose comes to the top and the fat remains on the bottom. When the lactose is removed, what remains is called ghee. Use it just like butter, to spread on toast or add to rice or vegetables. Ghee is never salted, so if you are spreading it on toast, you may want to add a touch of salt.

SUGAR—There are a few alternatives to raw sugar, however, they are mostly liquid, so swapping 1:1 is not the best strategy. For Type As, the best alternatives to sugar are blackstrap molasses, agave, maple syrup, maple sugar, and honey. Most of the recipes in this book call for agave and molasses because they are the most universally *Beneficial* sweeteners for the Blood Type Diet. You can experiment with swapping agave or molasses for a combination of the other sweeteners, however.

FLOUR—The best flours for baking are a combination for texture and taste. In this book we incorporate highly *Beneficial* flours. Although Type As can have whole wheat, try to use combinations such as spelt and oat; or oat, spelt, and buckwheat, because oat and buckwheat are *Beneficial* grains. Whole wheat can have a very earthy taste and hearty texture, whereas spelt and oat lend more of a tender softness that seems to be more appealing for most people.

A great everyday baking mix for Type A is:
>   2 parts spelt flour (⅔ cup for one batch)
>   1 part oat flour (⅓ cup for one batch)
>   Add 2 teaspoons baking powder and ½ teaspoon sea salt to
>   each batch.

Menu Planning

The following are suggestions to show you how to put the recipes in this book together to make weekly menus for you and your family. They are arranged in a way to keep a balanced diet, but feel free to mix and match as you see fit. If you plan to follow the menu exactly, read it thoroughly ahead of time so you can see where you would need to buy a little extra to account for leftovers, and where it would be practical to plan/prep ahead. The purpose of menu planning is to make life as easy as possible by utilizing leftovers and planning more involved meals for weekends.

In addition to the list below, make sure you are drinking a minimum of six (8-oz.) glasses of water per day to stay properly hydrated.

MENU PLANNING TIPS:
- If you work full-time or have difficulty preparing meals during the week, use a few hours on the weekend to prepare snacks and a few

meals for the week by pre-washing vegetables and lettuce. This will significantly cut down on weekday duties. A few foods that keep well and to have on hand: Flax Crackers, Granola, Spicy Nut Clusters, and occasionally Protein Bars.

■ If you don't like leftovers, it's time to start liking them. Leftovers are the most delightful time savers you could imagine. Pair them with a fresh salad or toss in a soup, and they will become your best friend, too.

■ When baking breads, muffins, or even sweet treats, freeze leftovers in sealable glass containers to keep them fresh. If you have Pumpkin Muffins in the freezer, you can pop them in the oven or toaster oven at 200 degrees for 10 to 15 minutes and they will be perfectly toasty and ready to eat.

■ When making something like bruschetta, double the topping recipe and reserve whatever is not used in a sealable glass container in the refrigerator for up to 1 week. That way you make it once and it can be used as many times as you want it.

Four-Week Meal Planner

Week 1

Sunday

BREAKFAST: Wild-Rice Waffles NS with blackberries and raw walnuts

LUNCH: Ratatouille NS

SNACK: Curried Egg Salad NS on celery sticks

DINNER: Turkey Chili Verde NS

Monday

BREAKFAST: Blackstrap-Cherry Granola NS, rice cereal, and almond milk with green tea and fresh blueberries

LUNCH: Leftover Turkey Chili Verde NS with mixed green salad dressed with lemon and olive oil

SNACK: Pear and Apple Chips NS and Rosemary-Nut Mix NS

DINNER: Lemon-Ginger Salmon NS with Brown Rice Salad NS

Tuesday

BREAKFAST: Scrambled Eggs with Blueberry-Macadamia Muffins NS and green tea

 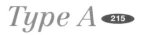

LUNCH: Raw Kale Salad with Zesty Lime Dressing NS and leftover
Lemon-Ginger Salmon NS

SNACK: Flax Crackers NS and Summer Squash Salsa NS

DINNER: Crispy-Coated Turkey Tenders with Apricot Dipping
Sauce NS and Pumpkin Ragu NS

Wednesday

BREAKFAST: Homemade Turkey Breakfast Sausage NS with green
tea and sliced mango

LUNCH: Raw Kale Salad with Zesty Lime Dressing NS and leftover
Crispy-Coated Turkey Tenders with Apricot Dipping Sauce NS

SNACK: Pear and Apple Chips NS and Rosemary-Nut Mix NS

DINNER: Grilled Radicchio and Walnut-Spinach Pesto NS

Thursday

BREAKFAST: Blueberry-Macadamia Muffins NS with leftover
Homemade Turkey Breakfast Sausage NS and green tea

LUNCH: Greens and Beans Salad NS

SNACK: Protein Blend™ Powder—Type A drink

DINNER: Tangy Pineapple and Tempeh Kabobs NS with Roasted
Autumn Roots NS

Friday

BREAKFAST: Quinoa Muesli NS, blueberries, and green tea

LUNCH: Leftover Greens and Beans Salad NS with feta cheese

SNACK: Carob–Walnut Butter–Stuffed Figs NS

DINNER: Mac and Cheese with Roasted Vegetables NS and Garlic–
Creamed Artichoke Spinach NS

Saturday

BREAKFAST: Broccoli Feta Frittata NS with green tea and pineapple

LUNCH: ½ Bacon Grilled Cheese NS with Roasted Parsnip Soup NS

SNACK: Peanut Butter Rice Cakes with Mini Chips NS

DINNER: Seafood Paella NS

Week 2

Sunday

BREAKFAST: Cherry Scones NS with almond butter and green tea

LUNCH: Fava Bean Stew NS

SNACK: Grilled Pineapple with Cinnamon Syrup NS

DINNER: Moroccan Tofu Tagine NS

Monday

BREAKFAST: Breakfast Egg Salad NS

LUNCH: Mint and Pumpkin Tabbouleh NS with leftover Moroccan Tofu Tagine NS

SNACK: Homemade Applesauce NS

DINNER: Shredded Turkey Bake NS

Tuesday

BREAKFAST: Quinoa Muesli NS with fresh blueberries

LUNCH: Leftover Shredded Turkey Bake NS with mixed greens dressed in olive oil and lemon

SNACK: Grilled Pineapple with Cinnamon Syrup NS

DINNER: Tofu and Shredded Escarole Soup NS and Red Quinoa–Mushroom Casserole NS

Wednesday

BREAKFAST: Turkey Bacon–Spinach Squares NS and green tea

LUNCH: Leftover Red Quinoa–Mushroom Casserole NS

SNACK: Cheese Toast NS

DINNER: Parchment-Baked Snapper NS

Thursday

BREAKFAST: Broccoli-Feta Frittata NS with green tea

LUNCH: Adzuki Hummus and Feta Sandwich NS

SNACK: Homemade Applesauce NS

DINNER: Rice and Bean Loaf NS with Bacon and Bean Collards NS

Friday

BREAKFAST: Granola–Nut Butter Fruit Slices NS with green tea

LUNCH: Rice and Bean Loaf NS sandwiches with sliced mozzarella cheese

SNACK: Protein Blend™ Powder—Type A drink

DINNER: Seafood Stew NS

Saturday

BREAKFAST: Pancakes NS with scrambled eggs and green tea

LUNCH: Salmon-Salad Radicchio Cups NS

SNACK: Crispy Spring Veggie Cakes NS
DINNER: Pumpkin Gnocchi with Basil-Cranberry Sauce NS with grilled chicken

Week 3

Sunday

BREAKFAST: Pear-Rosemary Bread NS with a poached egg and green tea

LUNCH: Fish Fillet Sandwich NS

SNACK: Crudités and Creamy Goat Cheese Dip NS

DINNER: Turkey Mole Drumsticks NS with Whipped Pumpkin Soufflé NS and Crunchy Kohlrabi Slaw NS

Monday

BREAKFAST: Creamy Peanut Butter Smoothie NS and green tea

LUNCH: Leftover Turkey Mole Drumsticks NS and Crunchy Kohlrabi Slaw NS

SNACK: Unibar® Protein Bar

DINNER: Salmon–Black Bean Cakes with Cilantro-Cream Sauce NS and Roasted Chestnuts and Rice NS

Tuesday

BREAKFAST: Pear-Rosemary Bread NS with scrambled eggs and green tea

LUNCH: Leftover Salmon–Black Bean Cakes with Cilantro-Cream Sauce NS with romaine dressed in lemon and olive oil

SNACK: Marinated Mozzarella NS with Flax Crackers NS

DINNER: Slow-Cooker Butternut Squash–Lentil Stew NS

Wednesday

BREAKFAST: Turkey Bacon–Spinach Squares NS and green tea

LUNCH: Leftover Slow-Cooker Butternut Squash–Lentil Stew NS

SNACK: Unibar® Protein Bar

DINNER: Broccoli–Northern Bean Soup NS with Green Tea–Poached Chicken NS

Thursday

BREAKFAST: Blackstrap-Cherry Granola NS, rice cereal, and almond milk with green tea and fresh blueberries

LUNCH: Shredded leftover Green Tea–Poached Chicken NS with cranberries and walnuts over spinach with olive oil and lemon

SNACK: Marinated Mozzarella NS with Flax Crackers NS

DINNER: Herb-Crusted Turkey Breast Stuffed with Shallots and Figs NS with Roasted Pumpkin with Fried Sage NS

Friday

BREAKFAST: Homemade Turkey Breakfast Sausage NS with green tea and sliced pineapple

LUNCH: Leftover Herb-Crusted Turkey Breast Stuffed with Shallots and Figs NS over Raw Kale Salad with Zesty Lime Dressing NS

SNACK: Unibar® Protein Bar

DINNER: Veggie Lasagna NS with Roasted Escarole NS

Saturday

BREAKFAST: Spinach and Zucchini Soufflé NS and green tea

LUNCH: Crunchy Kohlrabi Spring Rolls with Sweet Cherry Dip NS

SNACK: Farmer Cheese and Beet-Endive Cups NS

DINNER: Spring Pesto Pasta NS with grilled chicken

Week 4

Sunday

BREAKFAST: Savory Herb and Cheese Bread Pudding NS

LUNCH: Adzuki Hummus and Feta Sandwich NS

SNACK: Stone-Fruit Salad with Mint-Lime Dressing NS

DINNER: Shepherd's Pie topped with Roasted Garlic–Whipped Cauliflower NS with Roasted Escarole NS

Monday

BREAKFAST: Maple-Sausage Scramble NS and green tea

LUNCH: Leftover Shepherd's Pie topped with Roasted Garlic–Whipped Cauliflower NS

SNACK: Artichoke Bruschetta NS

DINNER: Seared Tuna with Fig and Basil Chutney NS and Herbed Quinoa NS

Tuesday

BREAKFAST: Pumpkin Muffins with Carob Drizzle NS with peanut butter and green tea

LUNCH: Baked Falafel NS

SNACK: Stone-Fruit Salad with Mint-Lime Dressing NS

DINNER: Bean Burgers NS and Broccolini Wrapped with Crispy Walnut Bacon NS

Wednesday

BREAKFAST: Granola–Nut Butter Fruit Slices NS with Tropical Kale Smoothie NS and green tea

LUNCH: Rotisserie chicken with leftover Broccolini Wrapped with Crispy Walnut Bacon NS

SNACK: Crudités and Creamy Goat Cheese Dip NS

DINNER: Ginger-Tofu Stir-Fry NS with Carrot-Ginger Soup NS

Thursday

BREAKFAST: Breakfast Egg Salad NS with green tea

LUNCH: Leftover Carrot-Ginger Soup NS and ½ Adzuki Hummus and Feta Sandwich NS

SNACK: Artichoke Bruschetta NS

DINNER: Pasta Carbonara with Crispy Kale NS with Greens and Beans Salad NS

Friday

BREAKFAST: Pumpkin Muffins with Carob Drizzle NS with peanut butter and green tea

LUNCH: Leftover Greens and Beans Salad NS with walnuts and fresh mozzarella cheese

SNACK: Crudités and Creamy Goat Cheese Dip NS and Adzuki Hummus NS

DINNER: Fish Tacos with Bean and Crunchy Fennel Slaw

Saturday

BREAKFAST: Cinnamon-Oat Crêpes NS and green tea

LUNCH: Melted Mozzarella–Onion Soup NS

SNACK: Baked Grapefruit with Honey and Cinnamon NS

DINNER: Chicken Pot Pie with Crunchy Topping NS

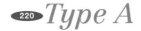

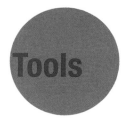

Tools

YOU CAN FIND the following helpful tools on our website at http://www.4yourtype.com/cookbooks.asp. You will be able to download these PDFs and print them from your computer.

- Food Journal
  Keep track of every meal with this handy log.

- Tracking Your Progress
  This is an additional tool to help you focus on your goals.

- Shopping List
  Make your shopping trip easy with this list of *Beneficial* foods for your type.

TYPE A SHOPPING LIST

Produce:

Artichokes	Lettuce	Blueberries
Broccoli	Onion	Cherries
Carrots	Pumpkin (when in	Figs
Celery	season)	Grapefruit
Fennel	Spinach	Pineapple
Kale	Apricots	

Baking:

Brown rice flour	Baking powder
Buckwheat flour	Sea salt
Oat flour	Agave
Spelt flour	Blackstrap molasses

Type A 221

Dairy:

Soy milk	Feta cheese	Ricotta
Eggs	Goat cheese	
Ghee	Mozzarella cheese	

Protein:

Tempeh	Turkey	Salmon
Tofu	Cod	Trout
Chicken	Red snapper	

Miscellaneous:

Olive oil	Adzuki beans	Ginger
Walnut oil	Black-eyed peas	Chamomile tea
Flaxseeds	Lentils	Coffee
Peanuts	Soybeans	Ginger tea
Peanut butter	Brown rice bread	Green tea
Pumpkin seeds	Soy sauce	Red wine
Walnuts	Garlic	

Please note: This shopping list only highlights the most frequently used *Beneficial* and some *Neutral* foods for Type A. For a complete list of *Beneficial*, *Neutral*, and *Avoids*, go to www.dadamo.com, *Eat Right 4 Your Type*, *Blood Type A Food, Beverage, and Supplement Lists,* or your SWAMI personalized nutrition plan.

Time to Think Green

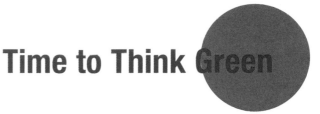

MICHEL NISCHAN IS a sustainable chef, cookbook author, and connoisseur of local, healthy food. He wrote in one of his books, *Sustainably Delicious: Making the World a Better Place, One Recipe at a Time*, "Where there is flavor, there are nutrients, and where there are nutrients, there is health." It is well known by chefs around the globe that the best food comes from the freshest ingredients, and nothing is fresher than a tomato grown in your own backyard or at the local farm. When I meander through my local farmers' market and browse fruits and vegetables picked at their peak of freshness, the smells, touch, and tastes become infinitely more vibrant than a similar stroll through the supermarket. If you start any meal with fresh, local, whole-food ingredients, almost anything you make will be the best-tasting food and the best for your health.

Here are a few highlights on buying organic, avoiding toxins in your kitchen, and shopping for the freshest fruits and vegetables.

Quick Review of the Terms

Whenever possible, buy organic food and grass-fed beef. Why? Conventional fruits and vegetables are sprayed with harmful chemicals such as herbicides, pesticides, and insecticides. The chemicals used in these substances can disrupt hormones, and potentially cause cancer, allergies, asthma, and other health issues. Meat, dairy, and poultry raised conventionally exist in poor conditions and are fed for the purpose of fast weight gain, which is taxing to their health. As a result, animals are given antibiotics that end up in the meat you buy at the grocery store. In addition, some animals are put on hormones to bulk up their bodies, making their meat artificially larger and, therefore, more desirable to consumers' eyes. Eating poultry is a *Neutral* source of food for Type As, but if the poultry is contaminated with hormones and antibiotics and causing unnecessary disruptions to your system, the goodness is essentially negated.

Here are a few definitions to sort out some of the confusion.

100 Percent USDA Certified Organic—This means that the product you purchase must contain ONLY organic ingredients, minus water and salt. Knowing the abbreviation USDA is an easy way to identify foods that are 100 percent certified organic.

Organic—Products must contain a minimum of 95 percent organic ingredients. Each ingredient within the product that is organic must also be labeled as such.

Made with Organic Ingredients—This label indicates that 70 percent or more ingredients in the product are organic. These products also cannot prominently display the word *organic*.

Natural—The product has to contain no artificial ingredients or added color and is processed in a way that does not fundamentally alter the product.

No Hormones—This term can only be used for beef. Poultry and pork are not allowed to be raised using hormones, so the label is unnecessary.

Grass-Fed—This term applies to animals that are solely fed grass and hay.

Free-Range—This indicates that animals are allowed access to the outside. This label is tricky, however, because there are a large number of farms that are keeping their animals in poor conditions but allowing a tiny space for "outdoor access" in order to be labeled "free-range." How do you determine if eggs are coming from humane farms? Check out http://www.cornucopia.org/organic-egg-scorecard/ for a scored list of farms.

Tips for Buying Local and Organic

Choosing Food That Is in Season

This phrase is tossed around a lot, but what is the benefit of eating in season? Taste. Obviously, it also has a significant environmental impact, but the difference between eating a fresh apple off a tree versus a genetically modified apple from the grocery store is striking enough to convince even the harshest skeptics. Eating in season also ensures that you are rotating the kinds of fruits and vegetables in your diet, and as a result, the nutrients. There is nothing more refreshing than fresh watermelon in the summer or roasted pumpkin in the fall. Make a habit of eating only the best by choosing local, organic food that is in season.

Where to Find Fresh Food in Season?

Look for local listings indicating farm stands or farmers markets. Most farms are also happy to show you around if you want to stop by for a visit or take your children to see how food is grown and raised. A terrific resource for finding local food is: www.localharvest.org. Just fill out your city/state and you will be provided with a listing of local and organic food happenings. Eating in season is more satisfying to the body and palate.

Local or Organic?

Sometimes we have to make the choice between eating local food or organic, and it can be confusing. Local food is terrific because of its freshness and limited impact on the environment; it does not have to be shipped all the way from Chile to get to your table. Food that is organic, however, is grown without harmful chemicals that are detrimental to your health but also negatively impact our environment. In an ideal world we wouldn't have to choose between organic and pesticide-free, but sometimes that is the choice we are faced with as consumers. Thankfully many independent local farms practice organic farming and this can limit the need for these choices.

Healthy Choices on a Budget

At some point, we all have to watch what we spend on everything, including food. The number-one tip for maintaining a healthy diet on a budget is prioritizing. If you are eating right for your blood type, you will be cutting out extras like potato chips, soda, prepared dips, cookies, and most overly processed foods. This alone will start to make room in your budget for healthier alternatives. Additionally, buying food in season is far less expensive than buying those same foods out of season. A pint of organic blueberries in the middle of the winter can cost up to $6.99; the same pint at the farmers market in the summer can go as low as $2.99. When stocking up on grains or nuts, be savvy and buy in bulk. Nuts contain fats that, if left in your pantry, could spoil quickly. To keep them fresh, store excess nuts in the freezer. Buying in bulk also means you are cutting down on the cost and waste of excess packaging, which you definitely pay for.

Finally, prioritizing your organic purchases will save you a bundle. There are twelve fruits and vegetables that carry the most pesticide residue; therefore, buying these ingredients organic should take priority. (See the foods on the Dirty Dozen listed below.) If you are on a budget, don't cut out these foods entirely, simply cut back how many you buy in one trip. Try to pick one or two ingredients that you must buy organic and supplement them with produce known to carry the lowest levels of pesticides, also known as the Clean Fifteen!

Dirty Dozen/Clean Fifteen

Below is a list of the Dirty Dozen. Try to buy these organic as often as possible to reduce your pesticide exposure.

1. Apples
2. Celery
3. Strawberries
4. Peaches
5. Spinach
6. Nectarines–imported
7. Grapes–imported
8. Sweet bell peppers (*Avoid* for A)
9. Potatoes (*Avoid* for A)
10. Blueberries—domestic
11. Lettuce
12. Kale/Collard greens

Listed here is the Clean Fifteen, a list of produce that has the smallest traces of pesticides and are therefore safest to buy in their conventional form. If it is possible, however, choosing organic is always better for yourself and the environment.

1. Onions
2. Sweet corn
3. Pineapples
4. Avocado
5. Asparagus
6. Sweet peas
7. Mangoes (*Avoid* for A)
8. Eggplant (*Avoid* for A)
9. Cantaloupe—domestic (*Avoid* for A)
10. Kiwi
11. Cabbage (*Avoid* for A)
12. Watermelon
13. Sweet potatoes
14. Grapefruit
15. Mushrooms

*Dirty Dozen and Clean Fifteen taken from the Environmental Working Group website, www.ewg.org.

Safe Food Storage

The first question is, what is safe? As most of us are aware, there is a chemical in most plastics called BPA (Biphenol-A), and when ingested it acts as a hormone disrupter. Studies recently conducted report that BPA negatively affects hormone levels, which can lead to obesity, as well as problems with thyroid function and certain cancers.

Where Is BPA Found?

BPA is a compound found in consumer products such as plastic containers, water bottles, plastic wrap, cans, and some cartons. Plastics labeled 3, 6, or 7 for recycling purposes often contain BPA.

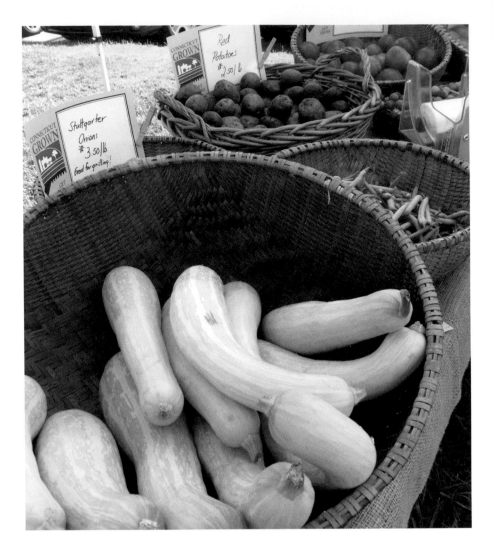

What Makes BPAs Leach into Our Food?

Cans contain BPA in their lining. Therefore, when a can contains foods
with high levels of acidity (like tomatoes), there is a greater likelihood that
BPA will seep into the food it contains. Foods with high acidity also affect
plastics, but a drastic change in the temperature of plastics (like freezing
or sitting in a warm car) will cause the same leaching effect.

How Do I Avoid Them?

Thankfully, it is getting easier and easier to avoid BPAs, mostly because
they are being banned by the government in most products for children.

Additionally, the more we know about the harmful effects of BPA, the more demand there is in the market for products that are free of this harmful chemical. There are many companies putting BPA-free products on the market. A terrific alternative to canned tomatoes are products packaged by Tetra Pak; all of their packaging is BPA-free. Additionally, look for foods packaged in glass jars as opposed to cans or plastics.

What Should Be Done About Buying Food in Plastic/Cans?

The best way to purchase food is fresh, in glass, or in Tetra Pak cartons. Meats and seafood that are packaged by your butcher in plastic can be swapped out at home for further storage. If you feel inclined, however, let your butcher know you would prefer your food wrapped in paper. If enough people speak up, a change will certainly happen.

How Do I Pack Safe School Lunches?

Traditionally, kids' lunch boxes and plastic bottles do contain BPAs. The good news is that there are an increasing number of BPA-free options available; you just have to look for them. Due to recent studies about the adverse affects of BPA on health, most companies are trying to or are required by law to switch to BPA-free packaging. That being said, glass containers with sealable lids are available in many different sizes and are another great alternative to plastic.

Get kids involved, so they start learning young. Let them help you in the process of preparing and packing their lunches. This allows them to learn about healthier nutrition. Choose fun, nontoxic snack packs for them to store their lunches.

Cleaning Up the Kitchen
What's Wrong with Chemicals?

Traditional household cleaners contain chemicals, such as alkylphenols, alkylphenol ethoxylates, ammonia, chlorine, and diethanolamine, just to name a few. These chemicals can cause allergies, skin irritation, asthma, and potentially much more serious health problems. Avoiding these chemicals and others in our environment is pretty much impossible, but what we can do is become aware of where they exist and limit our exposure as much as possible. The first step is cleaning out your detergents, bleach, disinfectant sprays, or wipes along with any other cleaning products.

Is It More Expensive to Use Natural Cleaners?

If you're smart about it, it doesn't have to be. In fact, cleaning with natural products can actually be less expensive. For example, vinegar is mentioned below as a replacement to some cleaning products. A generic brand of vinegar is about $0.02/ounce, and a little definitely goes a long way.

What Are Some Household Products That Can Clean Well?

The best non-toxic cleaners are vinegar, baking soda, lemon juice, and club soda. Vinegar is a natural disinfectant and believe it or not, deodorizer. You can use it to clean your floors, countertops, sinks, and any surface that needs cleaning. Baking soda mixed with water is slightly abrasive and can be used to clean stainless steel and carpets, and acts as a fabric softener and deodorizer.

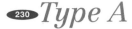

EAT RIGHT FOR YOUR TYPE PERSONALIZED COOKBOOK

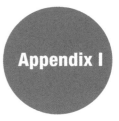

Additional Information on the Blood Type Diet

Discover Your Blood Type

It is difficult to begin a diet based on blood type if you are not aware of your own type. In Europe, blood type is something almost everyone knows, but here in the United States, unless we need a transfusion, we can go our entire lives without knowing what blood type we are. Here are several simple ways to find out your type:

Donate blood. Not only are you providing a critical service to the community, but this is a free and simple way to find out what blood type you are. To find your local donation center, visit the American Red Cross website's Give Blood page (www.redcrossblood.org).

Purchase a blood-typing test kit at D'Adamo Personalized Nutrition (www.4yourtype.com), under Books and Tests. The kit is inexpensive and simple to do in your own home.

Next time you visit your doctor for a blood workup, ask him or her to add blood type to the blood-draw protocol.

Secretor Status

We also address Secretor Status in this book, tagging each recipe to indicate if it is appropriate for both Secretors and Non-Secretors. If you do not know your Secretor Status, you can purchase a Secretor Status Test Kit from D'Adamo Personalized Nutrition (www.4yourtype.com).

Center of Excellence in Generative Medicine

The Center of Excellence (COE) in Generative Medicine is a collaboration between Dr. Peter D'Adamo and the University of Bridgeport to create a frontiers-focused biomedical initiative without parallel in any other medical school. The COE combines patient care, clinical research, and hands-on teaching opportunities for students in UB's Health Sciences program. It is also home to Dr. Peter D'Adamo's clinical practice. For information and appointments for either private practice patients or Clinic Shift patients, please contact:

Center of Excellence in Generative Medicine
115 Broad Street
Bridgeport, CT 06604
(203) 366-0526
www.generativemedicine.org/

D'Adamo Personalized Nutrition®—North American Pharmacal, Inc

For information on the Blood Type Diets, individualized supplements, and testing kits, please contact:

North American Pharmacal, Inc.
213 Danbury Road
Wilton, CT 06897
International: (203) 761-0042
Toll-Free USA: (877) 226-8973
Fax: (203) 761-0043
www.4yourtype.com

www.dadamo.com—For All Things Peter D'Adamo

One of the longest-running websites on the Internet, www.dadamo.com is the home page for the community of netizens who follow the work of Dr. Peter D'Adamo. This easy-to-navigate site is chock-full of helpful tools, blogs, and one of the warmest, most welcoming chat forums to be found. Newbies are welcome to this moderated, family-friendly community.

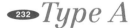

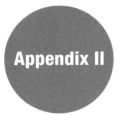

Dr. D'Adamo's products used in this book and where to find them:

Protein Blend™ Powder—Type A

Dr. D'Adamo created a specific protein powder to benefit the individual needs of each blood type. Type A has a high protein content based on rice protein and egg whites and contains no sugar.

Protein Blend™ Powder can be purchased online at: www.4yourtype .com. Simply click "Specialty Products" and scroll down to find Bars and Shakes.

Unibar® Protein Bar

The Unibar® is the healthy snack you don't have to feel guilty about! Designed by Dr. D'Adamo for all blood types, including Secretor and Non-Secretor, the Unibar® is ideal as a meal replacement, clean-fuel workout bar, or nutritious snack for a burst of energy between meals.

Chocolate-Cherry (15 grams of protein) and Blueberry-Almond (13 grams of protein) Unibars can be purchased online at: www.4yourtype .com. Simply click "Specialty Products" and scroll down to Bars and Shakes.

Carob Extract™

This delicious, irresistible syrup made from the carob bean is *Beneficial* for all blood types, for easing digestive discomfort as well as coping with fatigue. It's so good that 1 teaspoon a day won't be enough! Use as a topping on crêpes, ice cream, muffins, and even cereals.

Carob Extract can be purchased online at: www.4yourtype.com. Simply click "Specialty Products" and scroll down to find Bars and Shakes.

Proberry 3™ Liquid

Developed for immune support, Proberry 3™ comes in both capsules and liquid, but after tasting the liquid you will be hooked! I drink it by the teaspoonful when I have a cold, or drizzle it in smoothies, mix in ice cream, or stir into tea for a tasty boost of antioxidants.

Proberry 3™ can be purchased online at: www.4yourtype.com. Simply click "Right for All Types," then "Immune Support" and scroll down to find Proberry 3™ Liquid.

For a complete list of all products formulated by Dr. Peter J. D'Adamo, go to www.4yourtype.com.

SWAMI© Personalized Nutrition Software Program

Dr. D'Adamo developed the SWAMI software to harness the power of computers and artificial intelligence, using their tremendous precision and speed to help tailor unique one-of-a kind diets.

From its extensive knowledge base, SWAMI can evaluate more than 700 foods for more than 200 individual attributes (such as cholesterol level, gluten content, presence of antioxidants, etc.) to determine if that food is either a superfood or toxin for you. It provides a specific one-of-a-kind diet in an easy-to-read, friendly format. For more information about SWAMI, you can go to www.4yourtype.com.

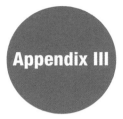

References

1. Bob's Red Mill. Bob's Red Mill Natural Foods. www.bobsredmill.com. Acccssed May 2013.

2. D'Adamo, Peter J., and Whitney, Catherine. *Eat Right 4 Your Blood Type*. New York: G. P. Putnam's Sons, 1996.

3. D'Adamo, Peter J., and Whitney, Catherine. *Live Right 4 Your Blood Type*. New York: G. P. Putnam's Sons, 2001.

4. "EWG's Shopper's Guide to Pesticides in Produce," Environmental Working Group. www.ewg.org, 2011.

5. "Food Labeling/Organic Foods," United States Department of Agriculture, www .usda.gov. Accessed May 2013.

6. Healthy Child Healthy World. www.healthychild.org. Accessed May 2013.

7. Mateljan, George. "The World's Healthiest Foods," www.whfoods.com. Accessed May 2013.

8. Nischan, Michel, and Goodbody, Mary. *Sustainably Delicious: Making the World a Better Place, One Recipe at a Time*. New York: Rodale Books, 2010.

Acknowledgments

PETER J. D'ADAMO

It is with great pleasure I share with the readers of *Eat Right 4 Your Type* and followers of my work on the Blood Type Diet my continuing explorations in the area of personalized medicine in the *Eat Right 4 Your Type Personalized Cookbook* series. There are many people I would like to thank, as this was a group effort.

My deep appreciation to Berkley Books, a division of Penguin Group (USA), as my longtime publisher; in particular, my editor, Denise Silvestro, whose personal belief in these cookbooks brought them from their original e-book format to where we are today; publisher, Leslie Gelbman; Allison Janice, who coordinated the production efforts; Pam Barricklow; the managing editor; and the entire Berkley team who worked on these books. I would also like to thank my dedicated agent, Janis Vallely, whose encouragement, guidance, and tenacity have made this book possible.

A very special thanks to Kristin O'Connor, whose culinary skills combined with her depth of knowledge of and belief in the Blood Type Diet, have allowed us to develop delicious, nutritious recipes that are right for your type.

A special nod of appreciation for our team at North American Pharmacal and Drum Hill, who worked on these books as they were being developed, especially Bob Messineo, Wendy Simmons-Taylor, Ann Quasarano, John Alvord, Emily D'Adamo, and Angela Bergamini.

As always, I am grateful to my wife and partner, Martha Mosko D'Adamo, for her unwavering support and for the role she played in shepherding these books into existence; and to my two daughters, Claudia and Emily, who share a deep passion for this work and for a well-cooked meal.

A final thanks to the hundreds of thousands of readers and followers who have shared this journey with me. I am encouraged and fortified by your continuing dedication to your personal health and well-being, and I am humbled by your trust and commitment to this work.

KRISTIN O'CONNOR

I am so fortunate to have such a huge arena of support; I truly could not have done it without any of you.

First, of course is Dr. Peter D'Adamo, the science behind this effective diet. I will always respect your brilliant mind and interest in making this world a healthier place. To my mother, Susan O'Connor, for being the reason I had so much faith in this diet, teaching me how to cook, supporting my every move, and being there by my side while testing all six hundred recipes! To my father, Kevin O'Connor, who sees more potential in me than anyone I've ever met, guided me in the basics of photography, and taught me to have the courage to put myself out there over and over again. My brother, Dr. Ryan O'Connor, for valuing my accomplishments and always sharing in the joy of my success as if it were his own . . . and being a very willing recipe-testing guinea pig! To my grandparents Mike and Ellie DeMaio, for being my cheerleaders, and for providing encouragement and unconditional support.

A huge thank you to David Domedion for utilizing his expertise to meticulously edit every recipe. Chris Bierlein for his incredible talent, kind spirit, and generosity with shooting and editing our gorgeous cover photos. We were privileged to work with both of you.

Heather Rahilly, whose friendship kept me sane and whose intellect kept me in the race, thank you for being the most thorough attorney I could ask for! To my friends, who are all like family to me, for selflessly offering help in any way they could: Annie Gaffron, Mandy Geisler, Latha Chirunomula (along with Padma and Pushpavathi for teaching me the basics of South Indian cooking), Jennifer Eastes, Iwona Lacka, and the Metwallys.

Thank you to Tim Macklin for being my very patient mentor, and a great source of knowledge and encouragement. Thanks to Danielle Boccher, Scott Olnhausen, and the rest of my pals at Concentric! Special thanks to Dr. Peter Bongiorno and Dr. Pina LoGiudice for taking me under their wing when I was just a little fledgling cook wanting to make a difference.

Thank you to Kate Fitzpatrick and Ann Quasarano, whose dependability and efforts at getting our book out there in the public eye was very much appreciated. To Stephen Czick for his hours of editing and support, and Wendy Simmons-Taylor for all her patience with styling these books.

Thanks to Martha D'Adamo and the team at Drum Hill Publishing for giving me the opportunity to work on these cookbooks, which I very much love and believe in.

And finally, a very special thank you to Craig Anderson for taking a chance on me at the very beginning and opening the doors to my dreams.

About the Authors

PETER J. D'ADAMO

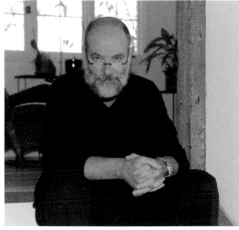

A second-generation naturopathic doctor, Dr. D'Adamo has been practicing naturopathic medicine for more than thirty years. Best known for his research on human blood groups and nutrition, Dr. D'Adamo is also a well-respected researcher in the field of natural products and a Distinguished Professor of Clinical Sciences at the University of Bridgeport. He is the founder and director of the Center of Excellence in Generative Medicine, a clinical, academic, and research institute, which also houses his private clinical practice, located in a beautifully restored Victorian house on the campus of the University of Bridgeport overlooking the Long Island Sound. Dr. D'Adamo is the recipient of the 1990 AANP Physician of the Year Award for his role in the creation of the *Journal of Naturopathic Medicine*.

Dr. D'Adamo's series of books are *New York Times* bestsellers and Book-of-the-Month Club selections. He was named the "Most Intriguing Health Author of 1999," and his first book, *Eat Right 4 Your Type*, was voted one of the "Ten Most Influential Health Books of All Time" by media industry analysts. *Publishers Weekly* called his third book, *Live Right 4 Your Type* "A comprehensive and fascinating theory that has been meticulously researched." His books have been translated into sixty-five languages, and there are over 7 million copies of his books worldwide.

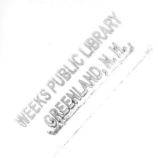

KRISTIN O'CONNOR

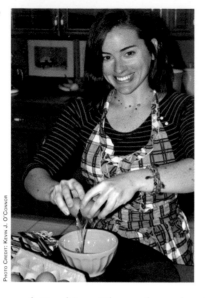

Photo Credit: Kevin J. O'Connor

Kristin O'Connor has made it her life's work to create food that is irresistibly tasty and healthy, a combination she hopes will inspire people to love good, healthy food and encourage them to make it a lifelong habit. In doing so, she created NourishThis.com—a website with recipes, articles, and tips on eating well and living green; volunteers for Healthy Child, Healthy World—a nonprofit that educates parents about nutritional and environmental issues affecting their children; and presented at the Kids Food Festival in Bryant Park, New York City. She has worked for a Food Network and Cooking Channel production company as an associate producer on many of their shows, was an above-the-line catering chef for a lead actor on a major motion picture, and is now working as a private celebrity chef. Kristin continues to volunteer for nonprofit organizations that promote a healthy diet and environment and hopes to continue her career as a cookbook author in the future.